Listening to Women After Childbirth

It is vital that healthcare practitioners understand the psychological impact of childbirth when caring for women. This accessible guide is designed to improve the care that women receive and, as a result, public health outcomes related to maternal and infant wellbeing.

This book outlines how clinicians can offer practical support to women after birth. It:

- discusses what we know about how women adapt to motherhood and develop a post-childbirth identity;
- outlines some of the causes and manifestations of post-traumatic stress following childbirth;
- provides practical guidance for setting up postnatal pathways for women traumatised by birth and how to communicate effectively;
- equips practitioners with the knowledge and skills to support pregnant women with a fear of birth;
- incorporates narratives from women to demonstrate how their births and related events were perceived and processed, before discussing how women's views can be used to inform future practice;
- highlights the importance of restorative supervision for healthcare professionals working in this area to promote staff resilience and sustainability.

Drawing together theoretical knowledge, evidence, practical skills and women's narratives to help clinicians understand the psychology of childbirth and support women, it is of significant value to all healthcare practitioners engaged in maternity services.

Alison Brodrick is a consultant midwife at Sheffield Teaching Hospitals, UK. Alison has established the Sheffield birth afterthoughts service and an antenatal service for pregnant women who are fearful of birth. She is also involved in service redesign within maternity.

Emma Williamson is a clinical psychologist at Sheffield Teaching Hospitals, UK. Emma currently works therapeutically with women who are experiencing symptoms of post-traumatic stress disorder following childbirth and has previously researched in this area.

Listening to Women After Childbirth

Alison Brodrick and Emma Williamson

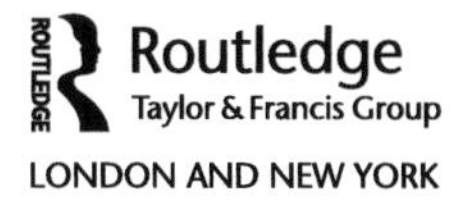

LONDON AND NEW YORK

First published 2020
by Routledge
2 Park Square, Milton Park, Abingdon, Oxon OX14 4RN

and by Routledge
52 Vanderbilt Avenue, New York, NY 10017

Routledge is an imprint of the Taylor & Francis Group, an informa business

British Library Cataloguing-in-Publication Data
A catalogue record for this book is available from the British Library

Library of Congress Cataloging-in-Publication Data
A catalog record has been requested for this book

ISBN: 978-0-8153-6033-9 (hbk)
ISBN: 978-0-8153-6035-3 (pbk)
ISBN: 978-1-351-11842-2 (ebk)

Typeset in Times New Roman
by Newgen Publishing UK

Contents

Boxes

Case studies

About the authors

Alison Brodrick RN RMDipHE MSc

Alison qualified as a midwife in 1994 and has worked in all areas of midwifery and in a variety of hospital and community settings but always with a clinical preference and keen interest in intrapartum care. Working as a consultant midwife for the NHS Institute for Innovation and Improvement from 2005 to 2010, she has a strong background in service improvement methodology and redesigning pathways of care. Since 2010 she has worked as a consultant midwife at Sheffield Teaching Hospitals NHS Trust with the most rewarding part of her job involving working with women to facilitate choice and supporting women who are fearful or anxious of birth. She set up the birth afterthoughts service in 2011 and works with a psychology team to deliver a birth trauma service. Research active, her interests are in women's experience of intrapartum care and fear of childbirth, and she has published widely.

Dr Emma Williamson BSc(Hons), DClinPsy, CPsychol

Emma qualified as a clinical psychologist in 2009. Throughout her career she has had an enduring interest in working with people who have experienced traumatic events, in a variety of contexts including health services and research. Since qualifying, she has worked as a clinical psychologist in hospital settings, including working therapeutically with women who are experiencing symptoms of post-traumatic stress disorder following childbirth. Emma has a particular interest in the interplay between trauma and attachment, specifically how a woman's own attachment style influences her response to a traumatic experience, and also how the experience of trauma affects her subsequent attachment to her infant. In addition she provides clinical supervision to midwives and nurses within the NHS, and strongly believes in the importance of psychological resilience in healthcare staff.

Foreword by Sheena Byrom OBE

The birth of a baby is the birth of a mother. How a woman journeys through pregnancy, labour and after the birth of her baby has the potential to significantly influence the way she adapts to her new role as a mother, her family relationships and her life in general. Childbirth matters – to individuals, to families, to parenting and future generations and to building cohesive societies. As maternity care workers strive to support childbearing women and their partners to maximise the opportunity for positive physical and psychological outcomes, they are often bombarded with challenges including workforce and environment constraints, facilitating the individual choices women make, and dealing with emotional and tangible traumatic events. If we want to improve the birth experience for women, we must also ensure that staff providing care are also cared for and supported, able to work cohesively within multi-disciplinary teams which place women and their families at the heart of service delivery.

Women are increasingly speaking out about their negative experience of childbirth. They are also expressing their fear of childbirth, even when they haven't yet given birth. At the same time, the explosion of media channels portraying negative accounts of childbirth and sometimes criticism of caregivers is influencing society in general, childbearing women and maternity services. The psychology of childbirth and motherhood is intricately woven throughout each woman's journey and through each narrative, shaping her beliefs her actions and ultimately her sense of self. This unique book, written by a consultant midwife and a psychologist, is timely and much needed. For anyone involved in maternity and psychology services the text offers theoretical underpinnings and evidence on why and how we should listen to women and act on their feedback to improve care. Poignant narratives of women bring the theory and evidence to life. The book is a fusion of psychology and midwifery with each informing the other. The psychology around normal cognitive and emotional adaptation post-birth that occurs as women process the experience of birth and motherhood is underpinned with practical information on how midwives in practice can support women who are distressed and how to recognise abnormal cognition and PTSD. Perspectives on the understanding and treatment of birth trauma are given, which can be used as a reference point for practitioners when planning care, or to support future research. The book is also important for childbirth activists, to help them to lobby for improved maternity services – to enhance the understanding that what happens to a mother when she gives birth matters to her and her baby in the long and short term.

Preface

Birth has the potential to be exciting, terrifying, beautiful, brutal – and is always profound. It can make a woman feel like a warrior or a goddess, or can leave her feeling angry, frightened and broken. The factors that make up the sum of a woman's birth experience are so varied and complex that we cannot give every woman her hoped-for birth, but we can ensure she feels supported, cared for, important and heard. Throughout history women have supported women through birth and the transition into motherhood, but the nature of birth and motherhood have changed in our modern world, and despite the deluge of information in our technological age, much of the inter-generational wisdom around this is now beyond some women's reach. Women go through so much to bring babies into the world, physically and emotionally, and they deserve to feel valued. The narratives used throughout this book are anonymous accounts, they are an accumulation of the stories and themes that we have heard reflected back over many years. We have written this book because women's experiences matter. Women's stories matter. Women matter. We owe them the time and the courage to hear what they have to say.

1 Transition to motherhood

Introduction

For some women, the transition to motherhood is a time of joy and happiness. The general view of the post-partum period within Western society is one of celebration, where mothers are in a blissful state of sleep-deprived gratitude for their new bundle of joy. In contrast to the image of total love and contentment encompassed within the 'Madonna myth' of mothering and motherhood, we are getting better at acknowledging that the reality may be quite different. Women describe various challenges during this period as they recover physically and emotionally from childbirth, often juggling additional responsibilities and adjusting to changes in relationships and family dynamics. It is a period of transition often accompanied by stress and a feeling of vulnerability (Mazzeschi et al, 2015).

It is estimated that 15–20 per cent of women will experience anxiety and depression in the first year after childbirth (NICE, 2014). In the last Confidential Enquiry into Maternal Deaths, suicide remains the leading cause of direct deaths occurring within a year after the end of pregnancy (Knight et al, 2017). Over the past few decades, there has been continual progress in promoting the understanding, assessment and treatment of the mental health difficulties that can affect women during pregnancy and the post-partum period. As a result, midwives, health visitors and GPs are more aware of the potential for women to be experiencing mental health problems around the birth of a child. Women are therefore more likely now to receive screening and support, particularly for postnatal depression (PND).

Psychological assessment, understanding and treatment have not, however, received the same level of attention. Back in 1996, Lesley Barclay and Beverley Lloyd raised concerns that an increased awareness and focus on diagnosing and treating PND leads to a risk of clinical depression becoming confused with the unhappiness, anxiety and frustration that many women feel after the birth of a baby (particularly for first-time mothers). They suggest that this potential over-diagnosis of PND is unhelpful in pathologising distress, as clinical depression may not be the most appropriate explanation for an emotional response which may actually be considered quite normal after the birth of a baby. Barclay and Lloyd (1996) describe a range of research showing that increased distress and lowered quality of life is in fact common and normal following childbirth, but for the majority of women, does not usually progress to a clinically significant depression. They conclude that the emphasis on providing psychiatric explanations for women's distress following childbirth ignores 'the possibility that women may be manifesting an appropriate response to the immense social, emotional and physical changes which they face in a culture that neither acknowledges nor sufficiently supports the process of becoming a mother' (1996, p. 138).

Within this context of normal elevations of distress, for women undergoing their first experience of birth, there is an additional psychological challenge: forming a new identity as a mother. As the philosopher Osho stated: 'the moment a child is born, the mother is also born. She never existed before. The woman existed, but the mother, never. A mother is something absolutely new.' For women having subsequent babies, the challenge may be different, but there will also be a period of emotional adjustment to being the mother of the new baby, as well as any existing children. Understanding these seismic changes in lifestyle, relationships, and even, or especially, sense of self is crucial to understanding how women recover from childbirth and to appreciate the additional effect and manifestation of birth trauma.

Becoming a mother: what happens

Back in 1967, Reva Rubin developed a theory of how women attain a sense of their 'maternal role'. She argued that women go through progressive stages in this process, beginning in pregnancy, where they will seek out information and expert 'role models', and fantasise about themselves as a mother. When a maternal role has been accomplished, Rubin said women feel a sense of 'being' in the role, and a comfort about their present and future. Rubin (1984) developed this theory further to acknowledge that motherhood is more than a role that can be inhabited and left; instead it is incorporated within the entire personality. Rubin went on to explain that certain 'tasks' are important in this process, beginning in pregnancy and lasting through the post-partum. These tasks include ensuring 'safe passage' and seeking acceptance for themselves and their baby, as well as a process of 'binding in' to the baby and the woman 'giving' of herself. Rubin also described how the development of this new dimension to a woman's personality is required with the birth not just of the woman's first child, but also of every subsequent child. As each baby is unique, so is the mother at that particular point in her life, and these 'tasks' must therefore be carried out to get to know and incorporate each child into her own self and family system.

Although getting to know one's baby and transitioning into this new identity is a time of often joyful growth and transformation, Rubin acknowledged that grief is also a normal part of this process. Women have to 'relinquish' parts of their lives which are incompatible with motherhood, and the nature and focus of this grief can be wide and varied. Many women experience feelings of loss around not having time for themselves, or for their relationships or other roles that had been important for them, as the needs of a baby are so initially all-consuming. Women may experience a feeling of loss as their previously held fantasy about what motherhood would feel like, or what kind of mother they may be, proves to be different to the reality. For some women, who may have consciously or unconsciously expected to experience the famous 'rush of love' for their infant, there may be a feeling of grief as they let go of this idea and adjust to what is the reality for many women, which more resembles a gradual process of falling in love.

Mercer (2004) advocates the use of the term 'Becoming a Mother' to describe what is happening to women following the birth of their first child. During Mercer's research, interviews and conversations with women about the experience of becoming a mother shed light on this process. Women talk about a sense of themselves needing to 'break' in order to remould their selves into a new identity that incorporates their baby, and their new caring role. For some women, this breaking process is experienced as painful, and is accompanied by a feeling of loss as women grieve for their previous selves and lives: amongst many others, women may miss their autonomy, their financial independence, spontaneity and time with their partner and friends.

Between 1943 and 1962, the influential paediatrician and psychoanalyst Donald Winnicott made approximately fifty BBC radio broadcasts on the subject of parenting. In these, he famously gave mothers compassionate and non-judgemental insights into parenting challenges and child behaviour. One of Winnicott's many contributions to understanding the subjective experience of mothers was to raise awareness of the idea that alongside the intense love a mother feels for her child, she will also inevitably at times feel much more negative towards them, and understandably so, given that 'he (the baby) is ruthless, treats her (the mother) as scum, an unpaid servant, a slave' (Winnicott, 1949, pp. 72–73). Winnicott explained that mothers tolerate these feelings without expressing them to their babies, and he expressed admiration for how mothers absorb so much hurt from their babies without 'paying the child out'. It is interesting that Winnicott not only saw these feelings of negativity as natural and inevitable, but he also believed they have a positive function in providing an environment where children can learn a full range and depth of emotional experience. Following on from this, psychotherapist and writer Rozsika Parker (1995) elaborated on the positive function of mothers experiencing both intense positive and negative feelings towards their babies in her book *Torn in Two: The Experience of Maternal Ambivalence*. Parker explained that when a mother can experience a full range of emotion in relation to her child, the child comes to learn that they have an impact on others, that they can hurt others but also repair relationships, and therefore they know themselves better. Seen through this lens, it is apparent that again, a rise in negative emotion and distress is a natural aspect of parenting, although one that many women find difficult and often shaming to become aware of, or own up to. This negative emotion, in conjunction with the potential for associated shame, becomes a further psychological challenge for women in the post-partum.

A woman's sense of becoming a mother is thought to be competency based; it gradually develops as women *do* more for their babies, and their confidence in their ability to perform the tasks of motherhood grows. It is interesting to note that our culture uses the term 'mother' both as a noun and a verb. We talk about 'mothering' as a behaviour, reflecting how this role is expressed in action. We know that the main facilitator of this process of learning to become a mother is social support. Women need to learn the skills of motherhood in order to care for their babies, but the act of this caring also serves to develop their competence as a mother, and consequently, their sense of self as a mother. Some of this learning may have happened implicitly over their lifetime: for many women, the skills of demonstrating care and nurture begin as a young girl playing with a doll. From early toddlerhood, some girls show a keen interest in babies and enjoy play that centres around providing care for dolls, imitating the mothering acts they may have experienced with their own caregiver. And of course, it is a girl's own mother (or mother-figure, if not the actual mother) who provides the first 'blueprint' or 'schema' of how to be a mother. It is through this mother, or mother-figure's actions that a girl begins to form an idea of what mothering looks and feels like. Clearly, these influences can be helpful or unhelpful in developing a woman's blueprint of motherhood. When unhelpful, these influences have been termed the 'ghosts in the nursery' (Fraiberg et al, 1975), referring to 'visitors from the unremembered past of the parents … [who] take up residence and conduct the rehearsal of the family tragedy from a tattered script' (pp. 387–388). A woman who grows up with a cold or critical mother may find herself unconsciously repeating this behaviour with her own children, or she may decide to reject this, banish the ghosts and give her own children a very different experience. A woman who, as a child, was made to eat everything, even food she detested, may overcompensate for this experience by deciding to take a very relaxed approach to food. She may also, however, not realise that she is passing on concerns about other aspects of her children's behaviour that she has internalised. This learning is life-long and is influenced by the mothers a woman is exposed to, whether they are real life mothers in her circle of family, friends and acquaintances, or the fantasy mothers she may come across in the media, or in literature. All of these sources build up a schema of what a mother does, what she looks like, and how she conducts herself in the world. Upon entering the realm of motherhood herself, a woman therefore has to negotiate her way through all of these influences to decide how the role of mother, and the act of mothering, fits with her own sense of self.

Beyond this very personal level of influence, women are also influenced by cultural ideas of how women ought to mother their children, and indeed, how mothers should behave in general. This can even influence a woman's feelings around how she ought to dress or wear her hair, in order to conform to, or again, reject the notion of what is culturally expected of her to do as a mother. This can feel like a tightrope for some women, not wanting to expose themselves to negative judgement from others for daring to dress in a way deemed to be sexy now they are mothers, but similarly, not wanting to attract the judgement of being 'mumsy', with all the negative connotations carried by that adjective. In her book, *Pretty Honest*, the writer Sali Hughes (2014) describes being visited by a friend when her eldest son was four weeks old. She reports picking what she felt was an appropriate outfit for the occasion, to demonstrate that she was coping well. Her friend, however, saw right through it, and it was Sali's choice of a pastel-coloured jumper after 'decades in heels, skinny jeans and killer make-up' that indicated to her friend that Sali was not feeling well, despite her efforts to 'look like a proper mum' (p. 239).

Even for women with much experience caring for babies within their own families and friendship circles, or professional experience if employed within a childcare setting, there is a significant difference between this and the continuous provision of care and feeling of ultimate responsibility for their own child. Much of the learning, therefore, must happen 'on the job', as women look to older, more experienced mothers, or health professionals, for guidance and tutoring in how to care for their babies. There is a general acknowledgement that the nature of this learning has changed in modern times. Previously, women would have received their informal tutoring in mothering skills from older female relatives, neighbours and friends. In our technology-savvy age, women increasingly turn to online resources and forums for their learning and advice and to maintain social connections with other mothers (Lupton, 2016). At the time of writing this chapter, entering 'how to' in the search bar of the Mumsnet generated 530,000 results, with topics as varied as how to unlatch a breastfeeding baby with teeth, how to keep laminate floors free of dust and how to update a CV after having children. Women continue to search for their answers of 'how to' perform the endlessly myriad tasks of motherhood as their identity as a mother continuously develops and evolves.

This idea of the self developing from a feeling of competency is important and relevant when considering women for whom birth has felt traumatic. For those women who feel let down and angry by those who were meant to care for them, their trust in their support system (both personal and/or professional) may have been broken to the extent that social support feels like a threat, rather than a source of strength and development. These women may then avoid seeking support because they have such limited trust that if they reach out, they will not find the support they need. For the many women who describe feeling that they have 'failed' if they were unable to have the labour and birth they had hoped for and planned, their journey into motherhood begins from a position of perceived inadequacy. Borrowing from Rubin's (1967) language, women may feel they were unable to provide the 'safe passage' for their baby which is one of the tasks of developing a maternal identity. Often, this starting point can be the beginning of a vicious cycle of perceived failures which only confirms a woman's beliefs that either professionals, or her very self, are not to be trusted. This process is illustrated in Dee's experience (see Case Study 1.1).

CASE STUDY 1.1 Dee's experience

Dee was in established labour when it was realised that her baby was in a breech position, and a decision was made to deliver the baby by emergency caesarean section at 11 o'clock at night. Dee had already been unwell with a chest infection when she went into labour, so during surgery she was placed on oxygen. This was left on until the following morning. Dee felt physically weak and overwhelmed by her physical symptoms and didn't have the energy to think about feeding her baby, which made her feel ashamed when she remembered this. That afternoon, a midwife on the ward suggested feeding the baby who struggled with latching on and became increasingly restless. Dee was also feeling unwell, and throughout the next night her screaming baby was taken away several times by the midwives and brought back calm and settled. Dee was confused and upset by this: why could they settle her baby and not her? Were they feeding her formula? The midwives denied giving the baby top-up feeds, but Dee began to feel that she could not trust them, and they must be lying. Dee found it hard to sleep because of her discomfort and coughing fits. Two other women in the bay began to complain that they couldn't get any rest 'with her making all that noise'. Dee felt angry and ashamed at this memory. She focused on being discharged from hospital, hoping that everything would resolve itself once she was at home with her baby in familiar surroundings, but to her dismay, the struggles with feeding continued once at home.

Despite seeking help from the community midwives and a local breastfeeding support group, the baby had lost 17 per cent of her birth weight by day ten, and the midwife worried she was becoming unresponsive. Again, this memory was full of shame for Dee. She and the baby were readmitted to the hospital, which recommended a regime of expressing milk and introduced regular formula feeds. This added to Dee's feelings of shame, and inadequacy. She also began to feel severe pain in her caesarean scar, and it was found that she had developed an infection. This made her feel more and more helpless and despairing of the situation, especially when the next day, some of her expressed milk was accidentally discarded. The feeding team visited her and said that there was no reason why she could not breastfeed her baby and that she just needed to persevere. A doctor told her, 'if you don't breastfeed, it will all be down to you.' She felt even more inadequate and could sense all of her confidence draining away. Eventually, she became frightened that the baby would lose more weight and that she would be referred to Social Services for neglecting her baby so gradually relied more and more on top-up formula feeds and attempted breastfeeding less and less, adding to her feelings of shame and inadequacy: she felt that she failed to give birth vaginally, and then failed to feed her baby. She was ashamed that her body could not do what it was supposed to do, and that she let her baby down. She felt she tried so hard to feed her baby in difficult circumstances, but professionals were cold and critical of her efforts, making her feel intimidated and threatened by people she had hoped would support and care for her. She could not enjoy getting to know her baby as she was constantly trying to feed or expressing milk. Dee looked back on her baby's birth with a sense of grief as she felt she missed out on those precious first days and weeks in a blur of illness, shame and fear.

Understanding the cultural context

When we expand our lens beyond the mother and her baby, we can see that mothers also exist within a wider social context, and this too has a powerful effect on her recovery from birth and adaptation to motherhood. Childbirth and motherhood are heavily laden with social judgements of what is deemed 'good' (Brauer, 2016). There are ongoing debates around what is considered the right way to deliver a baby, and what is the right way to then feed a baby, the right way to get a baby to sleep, and so on. These debates often become heated and emotive, with even women who do not subscribe to intensive, idealised ideologies about how to be 'the perfect mother' being at risk for increased anxiety and depression, and decreased self-efficacy associated with the pressure to be 'perfect' and guilt for not living up to high social expectations (Henderson et al, 2015). In the media, headline-grabbing, divisive debates use sexual politics to claim that women are either 'too posh to push' or have a right to not push and choose a planned caesarean section (Rustin, 2016). In maternity, this choice agenda is supported by the healthcare professionals, but only if it is considered the right choice; for instance if a woman chooses to give birth at home against recommended advice, some healthcare professionals deem this is as reckless behaviour and not the actions of a 'good mother' (Freely & Thomson, 2016; Miller, 2009).

Luce et al (2016) carried out a review of how childbirth is represented within the mass media. They discuss how women use portrayals of birth on television as preparation, but that the use of this medium as education is problematic because the dramatic portrayal of birth on television perpetuates the medicalisation of childbirth. This was supported by a content analysis of the popular reality television programme, 'One Born Every Minute', which also found an over-representation of medicalised birth (De Benedictis et al, 2019). This is despite some perceived cultural opinion promoting spontaneous non-medicalised births as being the ideal, leading some women to report feeling they have failed if they need analgesia or obstetric intervention. Brauer (2016) explained that favouring non-medicalised birth as the only way to find autonomy can put pressure on women who want or need anaesthesia and leave them feeling inferior and defective as well as ashamed: 'an anti-technological romanticism cannot be the standard' (p. 53). Within Luce et al's (2016) review, they found that the size and strength of opinion captured on the Internet creates a cultural ideal of what it means to be a good mother. With such strong and varied opinions on what is deemed acceptable and good within society, it is a confusing landscape for women to navigate in terms of how they come to evaluate their own experiences and choices.

Despite the prevalence of dramatic, medicalised births seen within the media, these are often coupled with a commonly held perception that a woman appraises any suffering she has endured as having 'all been worth it' for her baby, or that any pain and fear is instantly swept away by the rush of love she feels for her infant when it is placed in her arms. This is, of course, in contrast with the reality where many women do not feel an instant rush of love but take time to get to know and fall in love with their babies. While it may be some women's experience that any pain and fear they experience during birth is wiped out by the arrival of their baby, this is certainly not universal and for women who feel dissatisfied with their childbirth experience, the memory of pain is evident many years after the event (Waldenstrom & Schytt, 2009). Women feel a range of often conflicting emotions simultaneously. A loved and wanted baby does not always eliminate the distress endured during childbirth, and indeed, in our experience, for some women, can heighten it. Women who feel traumatised by childbirth often reveal their experience of bravely trying to share with others how they are truly feeling, only to be met by the well-meaning response 'but you have a healthy baby'. For the women we see, far from providing comfort, this comment often leaves women feeling guilt and shame about their emotional response and prevents them from seeking further support or help.

Some women who experience a birth that is very different from how they have hoped, or expected it would be, describe a sense of grief in response to this. The act of birth, and those early hours, days and weeks with a newborn are felt to be acutely fleeting, and impossible to get back once they are gone. When women feel this has been taken away from them, they may experience what is known as 'non-finite grief' – a term used to explain how we can grieve even when there has been no tangible loss. Women may not even realise they had hopes and fantasies about their birth experience until their reality is different and they are confronted with a painful discrepancy. An interesting study by De Groot and Vik (2017) included a thematic analysis of the comments on a Facebook post linked to an essay referring to a 'failed' birth plan. They called the loss of the dream birth experience a 'disenfranchised grief', which can be responded to in different ways: other people reinforce the sense of exclusion by processes such as 'one-upping' or are supportive through a sense of camaraderie and empathy. In our experience, the loss may be felt for the whole experience of birth, or for one of a myriad of aspects of the experience: women have described a sense of loss due to having a caesarean section, rather than a natural birth, for their baby being taken away for medical investigations after delivery and missing out on the 'golden hour' of bonding straight after birth, for being unable to give birth at home, or for many, many other reasons. In a model which has influenced traditional perspectives on grief counselling, grief has been described as 'work' by Worden (2008). He explained that there are four 'tasks' that a grieving person needs to complete in order to work through their grief, including accepting the reality of what has been lost, processing the pain of grief, adjusting and finding an enduring connection with what has been lost. When thinking about the losses a woman may feel as a result of her childbirth experience, these tasks do not easily fit: finding an enduring connection with what has been lost is challenging when it was not a material connection initially. A helpful alternative framework for understanding grief is the Dual Process Model of coping with bereavement by Stroebe and Schut (2010). This model posits that healthy grieving involves a process of oscillating between a 'loss-orientated' state, where grief may be intrusive, and a 'restoration-orientated' way of being, which is more focused on attending to life changes and developing new roles, identities and relationships. Oscillation between the two states is a necessary part of the grieving process, and another challenge for some women as they try to work through feelings of loss relating to birth experiences.

How we perceive events and the meaning we give to them can influence our ongoing sense of self in the form of the identity we are continuously developing. When considering a traumatic childbirth, it is clear that the way the birth is experienced and remembered can have significant implications for how a woman feels about that event, how she feels about herself as a mother, and how she feels about motherhood in general.

Autobiographical memory: how do we remember and how does this shape us?

Women report experiencing intense and mixed emotions during childbirth, with the potential for both positive and negative emotions to coexist. Childbirth can be experienced as joyful and terrifying, exciting and horrific, beautiful and brutal in rapid succession, or even seemingly simultaneously. Research has found that women use a combination of positive and negative adjectives to describe their experience, including 'exciting' and 'enjoyable' as well as 'difficult' and 'frightening' (Slade et al, 1993). This mixture of rapidly changing, intense emotions is illustrated in Mel's experience (see Case Study 1.2).

CASE STUDY 1.2 Mel's experience

At forty-one weeks pregnant, Mel went to bed one night with a restless feeling and struggled to sleep. She had some cramping pains but was not sure if they were the 'real thing' or a 'false alarm', which made her feel apprehensive. She felt frustrated at the sound of her partner snoring next to her. After a few hours, the cramping pains gradually intensified and she felt sure she was in labour, and so she woke her partner up. They started timing contractions and she felt excited that it was finally happening. Mel was pleased that she had taken some advice about coping with labour pain as she felt she was managing well with breathing, relaxation and getting into various positions to help herself feel more comfortable. Eventually, she began to feel the pain intensify and thought she might need to go to hospital; she felt terrified as they made their way to the labour ward in case she gave birth on the way, or in case they were turned away to go back home.

Mel was relieved to be admitted and a midwife helped her to settle into a room on the labour ward and made sure she was comfortable. Mel felt relaxed for a while as she was so pleased to be in hospital and felt safe. The midwife showed her how to use the gas and air and Mel felt pleased at how things were going. After a few more hours, Mel began to feel very tired and frustrated that nothing was happening. She sensed that the midwife was beginning to look concerned. She began to find it difficult to fully take in what was happening around her as she felt exhausted and the pain intensified. This was scary for her. She became aware of a doctor standing by her shoulder, explaining that her contractions had slowed down and they were a little concerned about the baby's heartbeat so would like to put her on a drip to 'give her a hand'. Mel felt frightened and vulnerable. Her contractions began to feel more intense again, and she felt overwhelmed by the physical sensations in her body.

When the midwife told her it was time to push, Mel felt that it would be impossible. In her mind she felt physically empty with nothing to give. The midwife and her partner were calm and encouraging and she focused all her strength on the sensation of pushing until her beautiful baby boy was born. When he was delivered, Mel felt utter panic, wanting to hear the midwife say that the child was alright: the midwife placed him on Mel's chest and she felt a unique combination of euphoric relief and utter exhaustion. The baby cried and Mel felt suddenly helpless, unsure what to do. The midwife gently advised Mel to talk to her baby and cuddle him, which she did. He calmed in her arms and she began to feel a glow of affection and pride.

Research tells us that the emotional content of an experience influences the way it is remembered (for example, see Hostler et al, 2018). The field of cognitive psychology has established that there are various types of memory systems within the brain, and emotion has the potential to interact with memory at every stage. During an experience, emotion will guide a person to direct their attention to salient aspects of what is going on. A woman in childbirth who is already feeling scared that something is wrong with her baby may therefore be focusing her attention more strongly on stimuli such as the sound of the heartbeat on the monitor, or the facial expressions of the health professionals in the room as she searches for clues as to what is going on. These stimuli are then more likely to be encoded into her memory and become more vivid parts of what she recalls about the experience. In contrast, a woman who is feeling relaxed is more likely to be attending to positive aspects of the experience, such as the supportive gestures of her partner, or the friendly warm manner of the midwife, and these become more encoded into her memory, influencing her remembering of the event in a positive way.

A woman's emotional state in the post-partum will also influence her memories of labour as when memories are being retrieved, emotion again plays a significant role. There is a broad range of evidence that our moods influence the nature of what we recall. Michael Natale and Michael Hantas (1982) carried out a classic experiment where they used a hypnotic mood-induction procedure with a sample of undergraduate students. Different mood states were provoked in the students, to feel either happy, sad or emotionally neutral. Inducing a sad mood caused the students to recall fewer positive life experiences, and also made it less likely that students could remember positive information about themselves. Inducing a happy mood, on the other hand, led to the opposite: students recalled fewer negative life events and more positive life events. This has been replicated in different settings since, and we can imagine how this is relevant when considering how a woman may be feeling about her experience of birth. If she is feeling overwhelmed by motherhood, it is likely she will be looking back on the labour and birth experience more negatively than if her adjustment to motherhood is going more smoothly.

The way in which we remember information is important because it is closely linked with our sense of self. The domain which is responsible for memory of events that we experience is referred to as 'autobiographical memory'. This is our memory system for who we are, containing information about ourselves, but also information about specific events in our lives. How childbirth is experienced emotionally is therefore important for the emotional valence of her memory of it, how that memory is encoded and retrieved, and for how she goes on to subsequently develop her sense of self as a mother. In addition, anxiety can significantly influence the recollection of previous experiences with anxious individuals more likely to remember threat-related stimuli and information (Mitte, 2008). Maternal anxiety during, or following childbirth will therefore affect not just the experience and memory of that event, but also has the potential to influence the way in which a woman adjusts to motherhood and develops her sense of maternal identity.

Maternal infant attachment

As well as the developing sense of self as a mother, another vital psychological process is occurring during pregnancy, birth and the post-partum: the developing attachment between the mother and the baby. This is also a crucial part of the context when a woman is trying to recover from a traumatic birth.

What is attachment?

The term 'attachment' refers to the close emotional bond that is formed between a baby and his or her caregiver (usually, and for the purpose of this book, the mother). It is characterised by a range of 'attachment behaviours' in both infants and caregivers. Babies will seek proximity to their attachment figure when they feel distressed, or experience distress when their attachment figure is absent. When caregivers respond to their babies sensitively and are 'tuned in' to their babies' emotional state, babies are able to form what is referred to as a 'secure attachment'. There is an immediate survival benefit to these behaviours in that the baby is motivated to stay close to their caregiver, and the caregiver can therefore provide protection and care. This synchronicity between the mother and baby, with both responding to one another's cues, can be observed even within the first minutes and hours of life (Malekpour, 2007).

Within this relationship and experience of being cared for, babies also learn that their needs are important, and they develop a basic sense of trust in others, and in the world around them, to meet their needs. This trust facilitates the baby developing the confidence to be able to reach out and explore their surroundings, with the mother as their 'safe base'. This can often be observed in the actions of a baby who has mastered the art of crawling, or in a toddler. They will often engage in periods of exploration or play, but will regularly crawl or toddle back to 'check in' with their mother, or read the expression on Mum's face for her approval that a particular thing is safe or acceptable to do. While this is obviously important for a baby's development in their very early life as they begin to learn about themselves, the world around them, and their relationships, it has also become apparent that this early experience actually establishes a 'blueprint' for the baby about how the world works, and how relationships are experienced, that continues to serve them throughout their lives. Since attachment theory was first developed by John Bowlby in 1958, there has been a growing body of evidence about the importance of the attachment relationship for a baby's ongoing social, emotional, physical and cognitive development.

In her book, *Why Love Matters*, Sue Gerhardt (2004) describes how 'the baby is an interactive project, not a self-powered one. The baby human organism has various systems ready to go, but many more that are incomplete and will only develop in response to other human input' (p. 18). Gerhardt goes on to explain that early experience has a great impact on the baby's physiological systems because these are in a delicate, unformed state in a baby's early life: 'Like a plant seedling, strong roots and good growth depend on environmental conditions, and this is most evident in the human infant's emotional capacities which are the least hard-wired in the animal kingdom, and the most influenced by experience' (2004, p. 19).

As explored earlier, cultural values will influence mothering behaviours, and will also therefore impact on the type of attachment that is formed. A culture which places a strong emphasis upon individual autonomy and independence may be more likely to result in different attachment relationships than a culture which prioritises interdependence and nurture. What is considered to be sensitive, responsive caregiving is a reflection upon the values and goals of that particular social environment and may differ between different cultural contexts (Rothbaum et al, 2000).

What influences attachment?

The advances in neuroscience that are detailed comprehensively in Gerhardt's book have shown us that early interactions between babies and their parents have lasting consequences.

These interactions are building and shaping the baby's nervous system and capacity for emotional regulation which go on to become core components of the future adult personality. Even within the 'nature versus nurture' debate, there is now more of a consensus that while we may be born with genetic predispositions and temperament, it is through our early relationships and interactions that these more 'hard-wired' factors are expressed. The way in which environmental factors (for example, social and cultural conditions as well as relationships) influences the expression of our genes is referred to as 'epigenetics'. Imagine, for example, a baby boy who seems to have a nervous temperament. Interactions which he perceives as critical of this aspect of himself – 'oh for goodness sake, get a grip, why are you worried about that, you silly boy' – will be experienced as shaming, placing further stress upon his ability to regulate his anxious response and either perpetuate the anxiety or, in line with cultural expectations about how a boy should feel and behave, he may learn to suppress his anxiety, leading to other difficulties then around acknowledging and expressing his full range of emotion. Interactions which may have sought to understand and help him to manage his anxieties – 'oh yes, I can see that is worrying for you, you can come and hold my hand and we'll face it together' – will instead help him, over time, to learn to recognise and cope with his anxious responses in a helpful way. As Lord Robert Winston, a professor and pioneer of fertility treatments, and Rebecca Chicot of The Essential Parenting Company explain: 'Imagine if the hugs, lullabies and smiles from parents could inoculate babies against heartbreak, adolescent angst and even help them pass their exams decades later. Well, evidence from the new branch of science called epigenetics is reporting that this long-term emotional inoculation might be possible' (2016, p. 12).

The ability to engage in this relationship of attachment behaviours relies on a caregiver's ability to be 'attuned' to the emotional state and needs of the baby. As we have seen above, a mother's own emotional state is going through significant upheaval, and providing this sensitive and responsive care for a baby can therefore be challenging. Luckily, the development of a secure attachment does not rely on the provision of perfect parenting, which is an unattainable goal. In his seminal book, *Playing and Reality*, Donald Winnicott (1971) spoke about the need to be a 'good enough' mother. He said that children need their mothers to fail them in tolerable ways so they can learn to live in an imperfect world. Normal life provides the mother and baby regular opportunity to experience this: every time a mother is not able to give the baby her undivided attention because she is tending to the needs of an older sibling, or the baby has to wait a few minutes to be fed while mother takes her coat off and has a much-needed trip to the loo, the baby is learning in small ways that life can be difficult, they will not always get what they want, but also that they will survive this frustration and disappointment. When a mother is also trying to emotionally recover from a traumatic birth, however, there is a significant additional challenge for them when also trying to provide this good enough mothering.

It is well established that the 'blueprint' for relationships that is established through these early attachment relationships go on to form the pattern for an individual's future adult relationships. John Bowlby, who initially developed the idea of attachment theory in the 1950s, described how this early attachment relationship becomes an 'internal working model' for future relationships. This is an idea which has been borne out by a vast array of research ever since, showing that our attachment style affects our romantic relationships, friendships, health, career and a range of other dimensions. As the psychologist Theodore Waters describes, 'there is a thread connecting life in your mother's arms and life in your lover's arms' (2004, p. 4).

In keeping with this idea of early attachment forming an 'internal working model' for future relationships, it is also known that people use healthcare professionals as attachment figures (Maunder & Hunter, 2016), and attachment style can influence the relationship a person develops with their healthcare providers. In 2013, Nynke Holwerda and colleagues looked at the relationship between patients and their doctors in the year following a cancer diagnosis, and found that securely attached patients felt more trusting of their doctors, and as a result, had greater satisfaction with their healthcare (Holwerda et al, 2013). While this has not been established in relation to a woman's relationships with her midwives, obstetricians, and other healthcare professionals during pregnancy and the post-partum, it is likely that this pattern holds true and may influence how a woman experiences her care and support during this time. Research has found that attachment style is a vulnerability factor for higher post-partum distress (including trauma), so there appear to be clinical implications for attachment style and the childbirth experience (Ayers et al, 2014).

Processing the birth during the post-partum: what is normal?

As we can see, a mother's brain is coping with a myriad of tasks following the birth of a baby, and doing so within a complex and sometimes confusing social environment. She is possibly experiencing some very normal and common elevations in distress as she constructs a new identity as a mother. Her hormonal milieu is adapting to post-partum changes and promoting the attachment processes described above. In addition, her brain is working hard to process the event of childbirth into her autobiographical memory in order to facilitate the developing sense of self as mother to the newborn.

Singer and Bluck (2001) discuss how people engage in 'narrative processing' of their life experiences, constructing stories of past events, ranging from brief anecdotes to more developed autobiographical accounts. They describe how people also engage in 'autobiographical reasoning': a process where people interpret and evaluate their memories, allowing them to make inferences and thematic links, and to learn lessons. In sum, people 'express their sense of self in stories, and these stories are important sources of self-definition' (2001, p. 92).

Anecdotally, post-partum women often want to talk about their experience of giving birth, with evidence that it allows women to makes sense of events and validate their experience (Baxter et al, 2014; Steele & Beadle, 2003). When we consider the importance of the narrative processing described above, it is no wonder that women seek out and seize opportunities to tell their birth story. In this way they are able to create a coherent and meaningful account of the birth within their autobiographical memory and develop their sense of self as a mother. Wang et al (2017, p. 199) describe narratives as 'a process of storytelling to reach a state of understanding' in line with an individual's cultural expectations. Their account states that this process of 'meaning-making' connects memory for personal experience and cultural influences within a framework of dynamic relations between culture, memory and narrative. Earlier in this chapter, we considered how our culture provides a confusing, contradictory and sometimes hostile context for women to experience birth. This makes it even more challenging for women to be engaging in this necessary task of developing their birth story.

A confusing and fragmented story full of trauma and fear is going to be a challenge to process, and potentially a negative influence on the emerging sense of maternal identity. This can fuel a need to seek out conversations with professionals to investigate their story, to fill in missing gaps in their memory, or to help them make sense of puzzling aspects of their memory, in order to achieve a coherent account. While doing so, she may be distressed as she processes the emotions as well as the events she has experienced. A meaningful and positive birth story, however, can provide a helpful launchpad from which a woman can go on to continue to develop her sense of self as a mother and enjoy the developing attachment with her baby.

Conclusion

When we view birth through a medical lens there is a risk that normal distress following birth is pathologised. The changes that we have described here, irrespective of a negative birth appraisal are likely to cause a degree of distress as a woman adapts to her new world. For most women the transition through instability, confusion and distress will eventually lead to a period of stability (Meleis et al, 2000). But this does not occur in a vacuum and does not occur instantly post-birth. For midwives and obstetricians working in a medical model, the challenge is to accept distress as a normative component of immediate post-partum care. When we start pathologising the woman who is upset and tearful by the recall of her birth events whilst still on the postnatal ward, we may further reinforce her belief of having failed when in fact she is behaving normally, allowing her brain to constructively ruminate and make sense of events. It is only later, as explained in Chapter 2, that we can identify clinically significant distressing responses. What women need in this early transition period is an empathic listener who can help her to make sense of her narrative and her emerging new identity.

References

Ayers, S., Jessop, D., Pike, A., Parfitt, Y. & Ford, E. (2014). The role of adult attachment style, birth intervention and support in posttraumatic stress after childbirth: A prospective study. *Journal of Affective Disorders*, 155, 295–298.

Barclay, L. M. & Lloyd, B. (1996). The misery of motherhood: Alternative approaches to maternal distress. *Midwifery,* 12(3), 136–139.

Baxter, J., McCourt, C. & Jarrett, P. (2014). What is current practice in offering debriefing services to post partum women and what are the perceptions of women in accessing these services: A critical review of the literature. *Midwifery*, 30(2), 194–219.

Bowlby, J. (1958). The nature of the child's tie to his mother. *International Journal of Psycho-Analysis*, 39, 350–373.

Brauer, S. (2016). Moral implications of obstetric technologies for pregnancy and motherhood. *Medicine Health Care and Philosophy,* 19(1), 45–54.

De Benedictis, S., Johnson, C., Roberts, J. & Spiby, H. (2019). Quantitative insights into televised birth: A content analysis of One Born Every Minute. *Critical Studies in Media Communication*, 36(1), 1–17.

De Groot, J. & Vik, T. (2017). Disenfranchised grief following a traumatic birth. *Journal of Loss and Trauma*, 22(4), 346–356.

Feeley, C. & Thomson, G. (2016). Tensions and conflicts in 'choice': Womens' experiences of freebirthing in the UK. Midwifery, 41, 16–21.

Fraiberg, S., Adelson, E. & Shapiro, V. (1975). Ghosts in the nursery: A psychoanalytic approach to the problems of impaired infant-mother relationships. *Journal of American Academy of Child Psychiatry,* 14(3), 387–421.

Gerhardt, S. (2004). *Why love matters: How affection shapes a baby's brain.* New York: Routledge/ Taylor & Francis Group.

Henderson, A., Harmon, S. & Newman, H. (2015). The price mothers pay, even when they are not buying it: Mental health consequences of idealised motherhood. *Sex Roles*, 74(12), 11–12.

Holwerda, N., Sanderman, R., Pool, G., Hinnen, C., Langendijk, J., Bemelman, W., Hagedoorn, M. & Sprangers, M. (2013). Do patients trust their physician? The role of attachment style in the patient-physician relationship within one year after a cancer diagnosis. *Acta Oncologica*, 52, 110–117.

Hostler, T., Wood, C. & Armitage, C. (2018). The influence of emotional cues on prospective memory: A systematic review with meta-analyses. *Cognition and Emotion*, 32(8), 1–19.

Hughes, S. (2014). *Pretty honest.* London: HarperCollins.

Knight, M., Nair, M., Tuffnell, D., Shakespeare, J., Kenyon, S. & Kurinczuk, J. J. (eds) on behalf of MBRRACE-UK. (2017). *Saving lives, improving mothers' care – Lessons learned to inform maternity care from the UK and Ireland Confidential Enquiries into Maternal Deaths and Morbidity 2013–15.* Oxford: National Perinatal Epidemiology Unit, University of Oxford.

Luce, A., Cash, M., Hundley, V., Cheyne, H., van Teijlingen, E. & Angell, C. (2016). "Is it realistic?" The portrayal of pregnancy and childbirth in the media. *BMC Pregnancy and Childbirth*, 16(1), 40.

Lupton (2016). The use and value of digital media for information about pregnancy and early motherhood: A focus group study. *BMC Pregnancy and Childbirth*, 16(1), 171.

Malekpour, M. (2007). Effects of attachment on early and later development. *British Journal of Developmental Disabilities*, 53(105), 81–95.

Maunder, R. & Hunter, J. (2016). Can patients be 'attached' to healthcare providers? An observational study to measure attachment phenomena in patient-provider relationships. *BMJ Open*. doi: 10.1136/bmjopen-2016–011068.

Mazzeschi, C., Pazzagli, C., Radi, G., Raspa, V. & Buratta, L. (2015). Antecedents of maternal parenting stress: The role of attachment style, prenatal attachment, and dyadic adjustment in first time mothers. *Frontiers in Psychology*, 6, 1–9.

Meleis, M. A. I., Sawyer, K. L., Im, K. E.-O., Hilfinger Messias, K. D. & Schumacher, K. K. (2000). Experiencing transitions: An emerging middle-range theory. *Advances in Nursing Science*, 23(1), 12–28.

Mercer, R. T. (2004). Becoming a mother versus maternal role attainment. *Journal of Nursing Scholarship*, 36(3), 226–232.

Miller, A. (2009). 'Midwife to myself': Birth narratives among women choosing unassisted homebirth. *Sociological Inquiry*, 79, 51–74.

Mitte, K. (2008). Memory bias for threatening information in anxiety and anxiety disorders: A meta-analytic review. *Psychological Bulletin*, 134(6), 886–911.

Natale, M. & Hantas, M. (1982). Effect of temporary mood states on selective memory about the self. *Journal of Personality and Social Psychology*, 42(5), 927–934.

National Institute for Health and Care Excellence (2014). *Antenatal and postnatal mental health: Clinical management and service guidance* [CG192]. London: National Institute for Health and Care Excellence.

Parker, R. (1995). *Torn in two: The experience of maternal ambivalence.* London: Virago.

Rothbaum, F., Weisz, J., Pott, M., Miyake, K. & Morelli, G. (2000). Attachment and culture: Security in the United States and Japan. *American Psychologist*, 55(10), 1093–1104.

Rubin, R. (1967). Attainment of the maternal role. Part 1: Processes. *Nursing Research*, 16(3), 237–245.

Rubin, R. (1984). *Maternal identity and the maternal experience.* New York: Springer.

Rustin, S. (2016). All British women have the right to a caesarean – they're not 'too posh to push'. *Guardian*, 29 March 2016. Available online: www.theguardian.com/commentisfree/2016/mar/29/british-women-right-caesarean-too-posh-to-push. [Accessed 4 November 2019].

Singer, J. & Bluck, S. (2001). New perspectives on autobiographical memory: The integration of narrative processing and autobiographical reasoning. *Review of General Psychology*, 5(2), 91–99.

Slade, P., MacPherson, S., Hume, A. & Maresh, M. (1993). Expectations, experiences and satisfaction with labour. *British Journal of Clinical Psychology*, 32(4), 469–483.

Steele, A. & Beadle, M. (2003). A survey of postnatal debriefing. *Journal of Advanced Nursing*, 43(2), 130–136.

Stroebe, M. & Schut, H. (2010). The dual process model of coping with bereavement: A decade on. *Omega*, 61(4), 273–289.

Waldenstrom, U. & Schytt, E. (2009). A longitudinal study of women's memory of labour pain – from 2 months to 5 years after the birth. *British Journal of Obstetrics and Gynaecology*, 116(4), 577–583.

Wang, Q., Song, Q. & Koh, J. (2017). Culture, memory, and narrative self-making. *Imagination, Cognition and Personality*, 37(2), 199–223.

Waters, T. (2004). Learning to love: From your mother's arms to your lover's arms. *The Medium (Voice of the University of Toronto),* 30(19), 1–4.

Winnicott, D. W. (1949). Hate in the counter-transference. *The International Journal of Psychoanalysis*, 30, 69–74.

Winnicott, D. (1971). *Playing and reality*. Oxford: Penguin.

Winston, R. & Chicot, R. (2016). The importance of early bonding on the long-term mental health and resilience of children. *London Journal of Primary Care*, 8(1), 12–14.

Worden, J. (2008). *Grief counselling and grief therapy: A handbook for the mental health practitioner* (4th edn). New York: Springer.

2 Post-traumatic stress disorder

Understanding the iceberg

Introduction

Post-traumatic stress disorder (PTSD) is a constellation of symptoms resulting in an individual feeling a sense of current, ongoing danger, despite the threatening trigger event being in the past. PTSD is rooted in the way in which the brain processes trauma, and has probably therefore been a human response to frightening events since the human brain evolved. As a clinical entity, PTSD was not formally identified until 1980 with much of the emerging evidence coming from observing war veterans throughout the conflicts of the twentieth century (Foy et al, 1984). These early incarnations of PTSD are well known to us through the terms 'shell shock' or 'combat fatigue' as it was recognised that huge numbers of war veterans seemed to suffer from a symptoms such as intrusive flashbacks, nightmares, excessive emotional reactions and hypervigilance, or a sense of being permanently 'on guard'. As PTSD began to be formally recognised, attention slowly shifted to understand how it can occur in populations other than military veterans, such as people who have been involved in natural disasters, accidents, or sexual violence. In was not until the 1990s that clinicians and researchers began talking about the possibility that the term 'birth trauma' may refer to more than just physical injury: childbirth – including 'normal' births – could also be psychologically traumatic and result in PTSD (for example, see Reynolds, 1997).

The current clinical framework for PTSD comes from the *Diagnostic and Statistical Manual for Mental Disorders* (DSM-5; American Psychiatric Association 2013), which provides the most widely accepted classification and criteria for diagnosing PTSD (see Box 2.1).

BOX 2.1 DSM-5 diagnostic criteria for post-traumatic stress disorder (PTSD)

A. Exposure to actual or threatened death, serious injury, or sexual violence in one (or more) of the following ways:
   1. Directly experiencing the traumatic events(s)
   2. Witnessing, in person, the event(s) as it occurred to others
   3. Learning that the traumatic event(s) occurred to a close family member or a close friend. In cases of actual or threatened death of a family member or friend, the event(s) must have been violent or accidental
   4. Experiencing repeated or extreme exposure to aversive details of the traumatic event(s) (e.g. first responders collecting human remains, police officers repeatedly exposed to details of child abuse)

B. Presence of one (or more) of the following intrusion symptoms associated with the traumatic event(s), beginning after the traumatic event(s) occurred:
   1. Recurrent, involuntary and intrusive distressing memories of the traumatic event(s)
   2. Recurrent distressing dreams in which the content and/or effect of the dream are related to the traumatic event(s)
   3. Dissociative reactions (e.g. flashbacks) in which the individual feels or acts as if the traumatic event were recurring
   4. Intense or prolonged psychological distress at exposure to internal or external cues that symbolise or resemble an aspect of the traumatic event(s)
   5. Marked physiological reactions to internal or external cues that symbolise or resemble an aspect of the traumatic event(s)

C. Persistent avoidance of stimuli associated with the traumatic event(s), beginning after the traumatic event(s) occurred, as evidenced by one or both of the following:
   1. Avoidance of or efforts to avoid distressing memories, thoughts or feelings about or closely associated with the traumatic event(s)
   2. Avoidance of or efforts to avoid external reminders (people, places, conversations, activities, objects, situations) that arouse distressing memories, thoughts or feelings about or closely associated with the traumatic event(s)

D. Negative alterations in cognitions and mood associated with the traumatic event(s), beginning or worsening after the traumatic event(s) occurred, as evidenced by two (or more) of the following:
   1. Inability to remember an important part of the traumatic event(s) (typically due to dissociative factors such as head injury, alcohol, or drugs)
   2. Persistent and exaggerated negative beliefs or expectations about oneself, others or the world (e.g. 'I am bad', 'No one can be trusted', 'The world is completely dangerous', 'My whole nervous system is permanently ruined')
   3. Persistent, distorted cognitions about the cause or consequences of the traumatic event(s) that lead the individual to blame himself/herself or others
   4. Persistent negative emotional state (e.g. fear, horror, anger, guilt or shame)
   5. Markedly diminished interest or participation in significant activities
   6. Feelings of detachment or estrangement from others
   7. Persistent inability to experience positive emotions (e.g. the inability to experience happiness, satisfaction, or loving feelings)

E. Marked alterations in arousal and reactivity associated with the traumatic event(s), beginning or worsening after the traumatic event(s) occurred, as evidenced by two (or more) of the following:
   1. Irritable behaviour and angry outbursts (with little or no provocation) typically expressed as verbal or physical aggression towards people or objects
   2. Reckless or self-destructive behaviour
   3. Hypervigilance
   4. Exaggerated startle response
   5. Problems with concentration
   6. Sleep disturbance (e.g. difficulty falling or staying asleep or restless sleep)

F. Duration of the disturbance (Criteria B, C, D and E) is more than one month

G. The disturbance causes clinically significant distress or impairment in social, occupational or other important areas of functioning

H. The disturbance is not attributable to the physiological effects of a substance (e.g. medication, alcohol) or another medical condition

PTSD and childbirth

A key understanding of PTSD is that it is not the nature of the event itself that defines it as traumatic, but the individual's subjective response to it: a person does not need to actually be in a life-threatening situation for their brain to perceive and react as if they were in one. This is important when we start to consider and address birth trauma.

Whilst studies have shown the existence of PTSD in pregnancy, these are often related to physical and/or sexual trauma (Loveland Cook et al, 2004), or high-risk pregnancy complications (Horsh et al, 2013). In the post-partum period the trauma is focused on the appraisal of the childbirth experience. As interest has grown in this area, studies have reported large variations in reported prevalence rates; a recent robust meta-analysis demonstrates a 4 per cent rate of PTSD following childbirth (Dikmen-Yildiz et al, 2017).

In addition, it is estimated that a further group of women experience clinically significant sub-threshold PTSD symptoms, which may not meet diagnostic criteria, but are of sufficient intensity to affect functioning and cause distress. Estimates for this group range from around 16 per cent (Dekel et al, 2017) up to around 30 per cent (Czarnocka & Slade, 2000; Olde et al, 2006). The variation in estimates of prevalence is thought to relate to the timing of assessment of the sample under study. It is common to experience post-traumatic stress symptoms in the immediate aftermath of a traumatic event as they relate to the brain's attempts to process and integrate the memories, but, for most people, these subside over time, with only a significant minority not experiencing a natural recovery (Dekel et al, 2017). Williams et al (2016) explain that some level of avoidance and intrusion symptoms are part of the normal adaptation following a traumatic event as the individual processes what has happened and attempts to adjust to their life following the trauma. Similarly, Slade (2006) points out that some measures of PTSD include items such as sleep disturbance and hypervigilance, which are normal, adaptive processes in the postnatal period as parents are providing round-the-clock care for a dependent newborn. It is therefore important not to pathologise early traumatic-stress-related symptoms, such as hypervigilance as they may actually represent helpful, required processes and behaviours in the post-partum period. In a study by Ayers et al (2015), hyperarousal symptoms were experienced by 50 per cent of women who had a non-traumatic birth.

Within the literature pertaining to PTSD in the general population, as well post-partum populations, the accepted time frame is the presence of symptoms for at least one month (DSM-5). It would appear that this time for natural recovery, together with the potential for heightened non-pathological symptoms, is even more crucial following birth. Prior to the one-month diagnostic cut-off point, an individual with PTSD symptoms may be considered to be suffering from acute stress disorder (see Box 2.2).

BOX 2.2 DSM-5 criteria for acute stress disorder

A. Exposure to actual or threatened death, serious injury, or sexual violence in one (or more) of the following ways:
   1. Directly experiencing the traumatic events(s)
   2. Witnessing, in person, the event(s) as it occurred to others
   3. Learning that the traumatic event(s) occurred to a close family member or a close friend. In cases of actual or threatened death of a family member or friend, the event(s) must have been violent or accidental

4. Experiencing repeated or extreme exposure to aversive details of the traumatic event(s) (e.g. first responders collecting human remains, police officers repeatedly exposed to details of child abuse)

B. Presence of nine (or more) of the following symptoms from any of the five categories of intrusion, negative mood, dissociation, avoidance, and arousal, beginning or worsening after the traumatic event(s) occurred:

1. Intrusion symptoms
   - Recurrent, involuntary, and intrusive distressing memories of the traumatic event(s). Note: In children, repetitive play may occur in which themes or aspects of the traumatic event(s) are expressed
   - Recurrent distressing dreams in which the content and/or effect of the dream are related to the events(s) Note: In children older than six years, there may be frightening dreams without recognisable content
   - Dissociative reactions (e.g., flashbacks) in which the individual feels or acts as if the traumatic event(s) were recurring. (Such reactions may occur on a continuum, with the most extreme expression being a complete loss of awareness of present surroundings.) Note: In children, trauma-specific reenactment may occur in play
   - Intense or prolonged psychological distress or marked physiological reactions in response to internal or external cues that symbolise or resemble an aspect of the traumatic events
2. Negative mood
   - Persistent inability to experience positive emotions (e.g. inability to experience happiness, satisfaction, or loving feelings)
3. Dissociative symptoms
   - An altered sense of the reality of one's surroundings or oneself (e.g. seeing oneself from another's perspective, being in a daze, time slowing)
   - Inability to remember an important aspect of the traumatic events(s) (typically due to dissociative amnesia and not to other factors such as head injury, alcohol, or drugs)
4. Avoidance symptoms
   - Efforts to avoid distressing memories, thoughts, or feelings about or closely associated with the traumatic event(s)
   - Efforts to avoid external reminders (people, places, conversations, activities, objects, situations) that arouse distressing memories, thoughts, or feelings about or closely associated with the traumatic event(s)
5. Arousal symptoms
   - Sleep disturbance (e.g. difficulty falling or staying asleep, restless sleep)
   - Irritable behaviour and angry outbursts (with little or no provocation) typically expressed as verbal or physical aggression towards people or objects
   - Hypervigilance
   - Problems with concentration
   - Exaggerated startle response

C. The duration of the disturbance (symptoms in Criterion B) is three days to one month after trauma exposure. Note: Symptoms typically begin immediately after the trauma, but persistence for at least three days and up to one month is needed to meet disorder criteria

D. The disturbance causes clinically significant distress or impairment in social, occupational, or other important areas of functioning
E. The disturbance is not attributable to the physiological effects of a substance (e.g. medication or alcohol) or other medical condition (e.g. mild traumatic brain injury) and is not better explained by brief psychotic disorder

While much can be learned from the general PTSD literature and considering how this applies to women following childbirth, there are many ways in which a traumatic experience of childbirth is different to other potentially traumatic events (McKenzie-Harg et al, 2015). As discussed in Chapter 1, positive social connotations of childbirth may make it difficult for a woman to admit to, or seek support for emotional distress relating to the birth of her baby, as the birth of a healthy baby is seen by society as a time for joy. Unlike most other trauma there is a need to consider at least two individuals at all times, mother and baby, plus a growing body of birth trauma relating to birth partners (for example, see Etheridge & Slade, 2017; Iles et al, 2011). Additionally the mother has to continue caring for her newborn baby, who may potentially serve as a reminder of the trauma and trigger re-experiencing symptoms. Finally, and importantly, unlike most other trauma the event of birth nearly always happens within the context of a formal caring relationship between the mother and her midwife or obstetrician. To feel traumatised when you considered yourself to be in the safe, compassionate hands of health professionals, carries a significant meaning that should not be underestimated.

As well as the direct impact on the mental health of the mother, it is crucial to understand, identify and address PTSD in mothers because of the potential consequences on the emerging relationship between the mother and baby. PTSD symptomatology has been found to be predictive of the mother–infant relationship (McDonald et al, 2011). This can have lasting consequences: PTSD in mothers has been shown to be potentially associated with babies' emotional regulation and increase their risk for mental health problems (for example, Bosquet-Enlow et al, 2011). It has also been shown that PTSD following childbirth can be associated with poor cognitive development well into the second year of life (Parfitt et al, 2013).

Understanding the symptomology of PTSD

The emergence of PTSD following childbirth can often be mistaken for the more commonly recognised post-partum mental health problem of post-natal depression (PND), partly due to the overlap in symptoms relating to a persistent negative emotional state and markedly diminished interest of participation in significant activities, both of which are key indicators of a depressive episode (see Box 2.3). PND is not seen as a separate diagnostic entity within the DSM-5, but is rather a specifier within the criterion for a major depressive disorder when the onset of the depressive episode has occurred within four weeks of childbirth. There is a general consensus in practice, however, that this is far too narrow and that depressive episodes within the first six to twelve months after giving birth should be considered PND. There is a high level of co-morbidity between PND and PTSD, with up to 72 per cent of women meeting criteria for post-partum PTSD also reporting PND (Dikmen-Yildiz et al, 2017). McKenzie-Harg et al (2015) suggest that in cases of co-morbidity, PND is usually secondary to PTSD. Treating PTSD should, for many women, lead to a resolution or alleviation of PND symptoms, although where PND is severe enough to affect motivation to engage with treatment, this may need attention first before PTSD symptoms can be addressed. Overall, it is important to understand and formulate the nature of a woman's distress and whether she is experiencing the specific elements of PTSD symptomology:

- Reliving
- Avoidance
- Hyperarousal

These symptoms presenting together in clusters are particular to PTSD, and less of a clinical feature within PND and, other psychological co-morbidities. There are clear differences in the diagnostic criteria of PTSD and PND, but also in their treatment and lived experience. Some women in our clinic have described the experience of misdiagnosis for their childbirth-related PTSD, being treated instead for PND with antidepressants, with no success. This sense of treatment failure can then compound existing feelings of hopelessness and negativity.

BOX 2.3 DSM-5 criteria for a major depressive episode

A. Five (or more) of the following symptoms have been present during the same two week period and represent a change from previous functioning; at least one of the symptoms is either (1) depressed mood or (2) loss of interest or pleasure. Note: do not include symptoms that are clearly due to a general medical condition, or mood-incongruent delusions or hallucinations
   1. Depressed mood most of the day, nearly every day, as indicated by either subjective report (e.g. feels sad or empty) or observation made by others (e.g. appears tearful). Note: in children and adolescents, can be irritable mood
   2. Markedly diminished interest or pleasure in all, or almost all, activities most of the day, nearly every day (as indicated by either subjective account or observation made by others)
   3. Significant weight loss when not dieting or weight gain (e.g. change of more than 5 per cent of body weight in a month) or decrease or increase in appetite nearly every day. Note: in children, consider failure to make expected weight gains)
   4. Insomnia or hypersomnia nearly every day.
   5. Psychomotor agitation or retardation nearly every day (observable by others, not merely subjective feelings of restlessness or being slowed down)
   6. Fatigue or loss of energy nearly every day
   7. Feelings of worthlessness or excessive or inappropriate guilt (which may be delusional) nearly every day (not merely self-reproach or guilt about being sick)
   8. Diminished ability to think or concentrate, or indecisiveness, nearly every day (either by subjective account or as observed by others)
   9. Recurrent thoughts of death (not just fear of dying), recurrent suicidal ideation without a specific plan, or a suicide attempt or a specific plan for committing suicide

B. The symptoms do not meet criteria for a mixed episode
C. The symptoms cause clinical significant distress or impairment in social, occupational, or other important areas of functioning
D. The symptoms are not due to the physiological effects of a substance (e.g. a drug of abuse, a medication) or a general medical condition (e.g. hypothyroidism)
E. The symptoms are not better accounted for by bereavement (i.e. after the loss of a loved one, the symptoms persist for longer than two months or are characterised by marked functional impairment, morbid preoccupation with worthlessness, suicidal ideation, psychotic symptoms, or psychomotor retardation)

Prevalence of co-morbidity with other psychological disorders such as post-partum psychosis and obsessive compulsive disorder (OCD) is yet to be established, although clinically there is some overlap in the presentations of these disorders. The compulsive ritualised behaviours seen within OCD, for example, can be a way in which women try to keep themselves and their babies safe in the face of the sense of the ongoing threat generated by PTSD. Similarly, some of the features of PTSD, including flashbacks and hypervigilance, share features with elements of psychotic symptoms including hallucinations and paranoia. Relationship difficulties are also a common consequence of childbirth-related PTSD for a variety of reasons; psychosexual issues can also arise due to avoidance of sex related to a fear of conception and the triggering of PTSD related memories (Elmir et al, 2010; French & Thompson, 2014).

Given the 'normal' nature of some of the symptoms of emotional distress seen in the postnatal period, and as discussed earlier, the warning not to over-pathologise (Barclay & Lloyd, 1996), it is challenging for clinicians to determine when a woman is experiencing distress related to the processing of the birth experience and adjustment to the postnatal period, and when their distress is more clinically significant and treatment is required. A useful rule of thumb is to refer back to the diagnostic criteria looking at whether or not the symptoms are causing clinically significant distress or causing impairment in important areas of functioning. Duration is another key indicator: many women experience fluctuations in mood during the postnatal period, but clinically significant disorders tend to be experienced in a more pervasive way (one month for PTSD; two weeks for a depressive episode).

To make sense of this complexity, it is useful to keep diagnostic criteria in mind, and consider these within a wider framework that allows for a thorough understanding of the different factors involved in a woman's presentation, but also the factors which were involved in the development of her symptoms, and those which are now maintaining them. Within psychological therapies, this understanding is referred to as a 'formulation', and, in essence, it seeks to explain what *has happened* for a woman, and what *is happening* for her now. This allows clinicians to ascertain the complexity of her presentation, without having to try to fit her symptoms neatly into a diagnostic box. It also shifts the focus away from pathologising the woman, with an implication that there is something wrong with her. Instead, the focus is on understanding her experiences and how they are affecting her now. Such a focus can then facilitate the clinician and the woman to work together to understand how to then intervene to alleviate symptoms and change unhelpful responses going forwards. This is explored further in Chapter 5.

Understanding trauma: what happens in the brain

For healthcare professionals caring for women post-partum, it is useful to understand how the brain is designed to deal with perceived threat and process traumatic experiences.

Understanding this in-built neurobiological mechanism, developed to facilitate our survival, helps us to understand why what may look like a 'traumatic' experience can be processed by women without resulting in psychological pathology.

In her book *Recovering from Trauma Using Compassion Focused Therapy* (2012), Clinical Psychologist Deborah Lee uses an analogy whereby different parts of the brain are imagined as characters with different jobs to do with processing threat and trauma. First, Lee describes the **thalamus** as having the role of 'gatekeeper', directing incoming stimuli to the applicable area of the brain. The stimuli may come into the brain through any of our five senses. Second, the **amygdala** acts as 'customs', checking through all incoming information for potential threats. Lee explains that the amygdala works as an alarm system in that it gives out surges of emotions in response to incoming stimuli, motivating us to take action if those stimuli are registered as a threat. The amygdala can be very sensitive and works on the principle of 'better safe than sorry'. The brain's priority is to keep us safe and to ensure our survival, so the amygdala's threshold for threat is therefore very low. Another feature of the amygdala is that it can reactivate bodily feelings and memories. It also creates associations between perceived threats and reminders of it, meaning that anything which reminds the amygdala of the threat will be perceived as a danger and responded to with the bodily feelings and memories from the time of the actual trauma.

Lee's third character is the **hippocampus**, which she terms the 'busy administrator', who, like a filing clerk, has the role of noting the times and places of events, and verifying the amygdala's assessment of threat. The hippocampus therefore has to cross-reference the threat to other memories held in the brain. When it decides there is no threat, the hippocampus sends a calming signal to the amygdala. When, on the other hand, a threat is confirmed, the whole brain creates a response to respond to the danger and ensure safety. Finally, the frontal cortex acts as the 'conductor' of the 'brain's emotional orchestra'. It facilitates and guides systems within the brain which regulate emotion, particularly the threat system.

These structures (or characters, to use Lee's analogy) comprise the 'threat protection system' (Gilbert, 2009). As we can see from the description above, its primary function is to protect us and promote our survival. For the woman who has experienced birth as traumatic, her amygdala will be highly sensitive, sending her signals relating to the threat and danger she is in, and as such, she may well present as very emotional and fearful. It is therefore important that the people around her, for example staff on the postnatal ward, are able to support the hippocampus and frontal cortex in calming the amygdala to allow for a natural resolution of the threat response. See Chapter 4 for a discussion on how this can be achieved by *defusing* emotional distress.

In addition to the threat protection system described above, our emotional regulation also relies on two further systems. The 'achieving and activating system' helps us to work towards our goals and achieve good things. The 'affiliative and soothing system' is linked to feelings of safeness and peace, with a sense of connection to others. It is thought that when our mental health is functioning well, these systems work together in balance: all three are necessary for our survival. Over, or under stimulation of these systems, however, can be problematic. When we focus too much on the achieving and activating system, for example, we become stuck in a state of wanting more and more, and not feeling satisfied. Similarly, if the 'affiliative and soothing' system is not activated sufficiently in childhood and our infantile distress is not consistently and adequately soothed, our brains will not learn how to readily activate this system for ourselves in adulthood and we may then struggle to experience feelings of love, kindness and warmth towards ourselves. It then becomes harder to call upon this system to balance out feelings of danger, and we therefore remain threat-focused.

How a woman perceives a threat to her, or her baby's safety during childbirth is therefore multi-faceted. Each woman has been uniquely shaped to respond to perceived threat, and how she is cared for during labour and in the post-partum will influence whether her threat and protection system is exacerbated or soothed.

Psychological models: understanding the formation and maintenance of PTSD

Over the past few decades, several theories and models of how PTSD develops have been proposed. As Grey (2007) explains, these models are not mutually exclusive but have differing emphases. Rooted in cognitive neuroscience, Brewin and colleagues developed the 'dual representation theory' of PTSD (Brewin et al, 1996; Brewin, 2003; and updated by Brewin et al, 2010), focusing on the nature of memory within PTSD. In this model, different memory systems within the brain are described to explain how normal, healthy memories are distinct to traumatic memories. Two main memory systems are proposed: contextual memory (akin to 'narrative' memory that is easily accessed in language) and low-level sensation-based memory that is perceived through senses. 'Healthy' memory relies on connection between these two memory domains, with interaction between narrative memory and sensation-based memory. In PTSD, it is thought that memory encoding involves relatively stronger sensation-based memory, weaker 'narrative' memory, and impaired connections between the two, resulting in a fragmented and disorganised overall recall of the event, with strong, vivid aspects of memory that can be experienced via reliving and flashbacks. A commonly seen example of this within our clinic is women describing an ongoing sense of feeling the canula in their hand, as this sensation has been encoded so strongly and not updated or elaborated by the narrative that would provide the awareness that this sensation belongs to an event in the past.

Ehlers and Clark (2000) developed a comprehensive cognitive model of PTSD that has strongly influenced therapeutic intervention and been shown to be a highly effective treatment (Ehlers et al, 2004). Their model proposes that PTSD symptoms arise as a result of a variety of processes leading to a sense of ongoing threat. For non-traumatic events, the brain processes the memory by integrating it into existing memories of the person's life story (the 'autobiographical memory base' referred to in Chapter 1). For a woman experiencing birth as non-traumatic, she will experience the birth as part of a continuous 'life story', with an ongoing sense of herself before, during and after the event.

Ehlers and Clark (2000) further suggest that trauma memories, in contrast, are not well elaborated, and are therefore poorly integrated with other autobiographical memories. Trauma memories do not have a 'time-code', so when they are triggered, they feel like something that is happening in the here and now, rather than being something from the past. The memories are readily triggered due to being so poorly elaborated within the memory system, as seen in Evie's experience (Case Study 2.1).

CASE STUDY 2.1 Evie's experience

Evie struggled with flashbacks of her emergency caesarean section, which were triggered by switching on her bathroom light. The luminosity of the bathroom light matched a sensory memory of the lights in theatre, and as a result, she felt the same rush of fear and panic she had felt at the time she was wheeled into theatre.

Negative appraisals

Throughout various understandings of PTSD, it is seen that the *meaning* that a person makes of their traumatic experience and any subsequent symptoms will influence how it is processed and experienced on an emotional level. In their model, Ehlers and Clark (2000) describe how negative appraisals of the traumatic event, its sequalae and any emerging PTSD symptoms serve to maintain and strengthen the sense of threat. Subsequent models of PTSD have built upon this idea, with Bennett & Wells (2010) describing the role of 'meta-cognition' in the development of PTSD symptoms. Their research identified that a person's *beliefs* about their trauma memories were linked to PTSD, rather than characteristics of the memory itself. This is consistent with what we know about emotional memory in general, not just traumatic memories. Emotional regulation strategies, such as the reappraisal of an event, influence the nature of how that event is remembered, and subsequent mood (Denkova et al, 2012).

This has also been found to be relevant for the appraisals women make during and after childbirth, with meta-cognition being thought to play a key role in the development of post-partum psychological distress (Williams et al, 2016). Dekel et al (2017) carried out a systematic review which found that a negative subjective experience of childbirth is the most potent predictor of PTSD, particularly when women have feared for themselves or their baby during the birth, and felt a low sense of control. Dekel et al (2017) categorise two types of negative appraisal in their review: appraisals of the event itself (which they term the 'primary appraisal') and of their ability to cope ('secondary appraisal'). As healthcare professionals, it is important to remember that it is this subjective appraisal which matters to the woman even when from a clinician perspective the events appear undramatic and free of danger. For instance a common narrative from women is their interpretation of newborn infant resuscitation. In Clare's narrative (Case Study 2.2), she remembers being told that she had to push harder and that her baby was 'not happy' and needed to be delivered now. Her baby was born with the aid of a ventouse and until she came to a birth afterthoughts session to talk through her birth with a midwife believed that her failure to push hard enough resulted in her baby's condition at birth which she interpreted as 'nearly died'.

CASE STUDY 2.2 Clare's experience

'It felt like they were pulling a rabbit from a hat, only he was lifeless, blue, not moving, I thought I have done this, it's my fault, everyone was crowded around him, no one spoke to us and I don't know how long it was before he cried, then they put him on me and I just felt numb.'

In this scenario, Clare believes at the moment of birth that her baby is dead. Women often believe that if the baby is not breathing then the heart must have also stopped. This is rarely the case in this type of scenario, yet outside of obstetrics the mechanism of newborn adaptation is unlikely to be well known. Clare's emotional response therefore is fear and guilt, resulting in her threat system being alerted, and memories are encoded in the sensory, fragmented way described above. In fact, the baby required no other support other than the usual rub down with a towel, and inflation breaths, an extremely common occurrence on the labour ward. Breathing was established by one minute, followed by a cry. We often find that when this is explained, alongside the normal physiology of a newborn needing to adjust to breathing in dry air, the common response is 'but no one has explained that before'.

Offered a new perspective, Clare was able to explore and adapt her negative cognition. It is interesting to note that in this scenario it was actually her birth partner (husband) who was most traumatised; he was unable to talk about the birth and did not accompany Clare to birth afterthoughts. He accessed talking therapies through his GP and came back to birth afterthoughts some 10 months after the birth as this was the first time he felt able to re-experience the birth and to understand about the actual events at the time of birth.

Case Study 2.3 describes Jenny's experience. Sadly, Jenny did not receive the new perspective to her negative cognitions that Clare benefitted from, and we see from her experience how this has ongoing consequences.

CASE STUDY 2.3 Jenny's experience

Jenny had a long labour with her first baby, and she had to use all of her strength to cope with the pain of the intense contractions. She could see that her partner felt helpless, and she felt guilty that her partner was feeling that way. She felt that her midwife wasn't really interested in looking after her as she seemed quite 'hands off', and Jenny felt at a loss to know how to manage the process better. She was usually such a perfectionist and it seemed strange and frustrating to her that she was finding labour so hard. The pushing stage seemed to take forever. Jenny felt she was putting all of her strength into each push and began to feel despairing that there seemed to be no progress. Eventually, after some time and some examinations, a doctor told Jenny that 'due to lack of maternal effort' they would have to deliver the baby via forceps. Jenny was terrified as they rushed her into theatre for the procedure, and she saw a look of panic on her partner's face. She felt guilty that she was putting her partner and baby through such an ordeal because of her 'lack of effort'. She felt fear too, that there would be something wrong with the baby, or that the forceps would injure her or the baby. She had a friend of a friend whose baby's eyesight was damaged by a forceps delivery. When the baby was born, and everything seemed OK, Jenny felt relieved at first, but after a few hours, she began to think about what had happened. The phrase 'lack of maternal effort' kept going around in her mind. When her mum came to the ward later that day to meet the baby, Jenny and her partner were describing the birth. Jenny's partner said, 'Jenny tried really hard but it wasn't enough, so they used forceps.' This felt crushing for Jenny as it confirmed the fear that had been growing in her since the delivery, that she was a failure, she had been weak and inadequate as a woman. A cloud of shame came over her. Jenny was discharged home the next day and could not stop thinking about the birth, particularly the comment about 'lack of effort', the look of panic on her partner's face and the feeling of terror that she had experienced.

Over the next few weeks, Jenny hoped she would start feeling better but found herself ruminating more and more. She believed that because she had been such a failure and unable to push her baby out unaided, she was also going to be a failure as a mother. She became acutely aware of any signs of a bond between them, and as her baby began being more responsive, Jenny decided that her baby did not love her at all, and showed a preference for her partner and grandparents. This triggered further panic in Jenny, and she became very possessive of her baby. The idea of someone else holding, or worse still, looking after her baby, became very anxiety-provoking. Jenny found the thought that she had been cut during the episiotomy disgusting and believed that her body had been ruined. She distanced herself from her partner out of fear that he too would find her body disgusting. She found it difficult to sleep, even when her baby was sleeping, and when she did sleep, she had recurrent nightmares about births, where she would deliver multiple deformed babies. Thinking about the birth also brought up memories from Jenny's past, and she found herself remembering her childhood when she had been bullied.

Jenny avoided seeing people because she didn't want them to ask about the birth, and for her to have to tell them she had been such a failure. She avoided talking or thinking about births in general, her own, or anyone else's. She hated seeing other babies or pregnant women as this made her relive her own experience, but also made her feel more ashamed: why could they cope so well, and be so happy, when she was finding it all so difficult?

Jenny felt as if nobody could understand. Her health visitor told her she was depressed, but Jenny had suffered from depression in the past and she knew this felt different. She was overwhelmed by shame about the birth, about her body, about the lack of bond she perceived between herself and her baby, about not having 'got over it' yet. Jenny was on edge, and lived in fear that someone else would see her for the inadequate and disgusting person she believed herself to be.

Pre- and peri-traumatic factors

As well as the model described above by Ehlers and Clark (2000), additional factors involved in processing trauma include pre-traumatic factors, such as-prior experience, personality and coping style of the individual, and peri-traumatic factors relating to the labour experience. Various studies have examined pre-birth characteristics and factors which are associated with subsequent development of PTSD in order to help clinicians to identify which women may be more at risk. Ayers (2004) found that a prior experience of PTSD is a significant vulnerability factor for childbirth-related PTSD because existing symptoms interact with birth events to generate an appraisal of the birth as traumatic, and this can then influence the development of traumatic stress responses. A systematic review by Dekel et al (2017) found that previous trauma exposure is also important in the development of PTSD following childbirth, especially childhood sexual trauma, interpersonal violence and a previous traumatic birth experience. Dekel et al (2017) also identified demographic risk factors including young age and low income being more highly associated with the development of PTSD following birth. Ayers et al (2016) found that depression in pregnancy is a key risk factor, along with fear of childbirth, poor health or complications in pregnancy, a history of PTSD or counselling for pregnancy or birth related factors. Ayers et al (2016) suggested that there may be differences in some risk factors between low and middle income countries and high income countries, which they speculate may be related to different rates of maternal morbidity and mortality in these countries.

Obstetric peri-traumatic factors associated with PTSD, include delivery by emergency caesarean section, complications with the pregnancy and/or baby, and instrumental deliveries (Dekel et al, 2017). Infant complications including pre-term labour, newborn birth asphyxia, low birthweight and the infant developing medical complications and/or a handicap have also been identified (Andersen et al, 2012).

What is significant in Dekel et al's (2017) systematic review is that risk factors related to the delivery mode and complications in labour were only the fourth highest predictive category behind negative subjective experience, maternal mental health and trauma history. Negative subjective birth experience has consistently been found to be the strongest risk factor for PTSD (Ayers et al, 2016; Andersen et al, 2012) as has a lack of support during the birth and dissatisfaction with health professionals (Ayers et al, 2016; Dikmen-Yildiz et al, 2017; Harris & Ayers, 2012). Whilst studies have shown some correlation between obstetric complications and PTSD, it cannot be used as a reliable predictor of PTSD developing for a woman.

Perinatal negative emotional reactions and perinatal dissociative reactions have also been shown to be predictive of PTSD symptoms (Olde et al, 2005). Dissociation is a psychological phenomenon whereby a person finds themselves feeling detached from themselves and their emotions, perhaps with a perception of stimuli around them seeming unreal. This can be in the form of an out-of-body experience, a temporal coping mechanism which women describe as floating above the scene or separation of a body part from the main body (Bateman et al, 2017). It may also be accompanied by memory loss. Olde et al (2005) studied this phenomenon in relation to childbirth because it had been shown to be a significant predictor of trauma in the general literature. They found that women who experienced an instrumental delivery and reported high levels of dissociation were at higher risk of developing PTSD than women who described high levels of dissociation during a spontaneous delivery.

See Case Study 2.4 for a description of Sarah's narrative. Sarah self-referred to birth afterthoughts eight months after the birth of her first child. She was experiencing frequent intrusive memories of the birth, associated with a sense of panic, and was coping by trying to avoid all reminders of it, a particularly problematic strategy as she was a midwife. Sarah knew that she needed help to emotionally reconcile her journey and to be able to help women in labour without being overwhelmed by her own memories and emotions. Following the birth afterthoughts session, she was referred for psychology input and has since returned to work, where she says she has new-found skills and confidence in supporting women with their emotional response to their childbirth experience in the post-partum.

CASE STUDY 2.4 Sarah's experience

'… I had lost it, I just wanted her to be taken out but I was still in midwife mode, not wanting to be the difficult patient, I remember looking intently at my partner and willing him to understand that I needed help, to understand that I needed help, I could do no more, I didn't speak to anyone, I didn't tell them how I felt, I just wanted someone to help me, to realise what I was going through but no one responded. I didn't care when he [doctor] said he could help me with a lift out, I made a joke I think, I just wanted it to be over … I can remember looking down from the ceiling and I can see him do the episiotomy, I watched it from above, I know rationally that this is not possible, but I have this image of being above myself and seeing him cut me … I can't get rid of it.'

In Sarah's case, she describes feeling helpless and abandoned by her partner and the staff. Although logically she realised that she didn't articulate that she needed help, a rational understanding does not always dissipate the anxiety and fear that accompanies the experience. These unresolved emotions led to a frequent re-experiencing of events and revisiting the scene from her viewpoint of being on the ceiling.

Overwhelmingly, whilst multiple risk factors have been reported, the cumulative evidence around pre and peri-traumatic factors in relation to childbirth is consistent in the assertion that how a woman subjectively experiences the birth is the crucial factor in how she goes on to process and adapt to her memories of it.

Post-traumatic factors

Following a traumatic event, it is common for women to try and manage the resulting emotional stress by adopting strategies that may exacerbate and maintain the distress by blocking the processing that allows the necessary integration of the event into memory (Ehlers & Clark, 2000). Such strategies often include avoidance of reminders of the event. A common narrative from women is the inability to look at any photographs of their baby as a newborn and especially photos taken just after birth. Hospital bags too may remain unpacked for many months, or items used at the time of the birth may be discarded to avoid the memories they trigger.

The therapeutic intervention of 'reliving' or exposure to the trauma memory is often used in the treatment of PTSD, to overcome this reflex of avoidance and facilitate the processing and elaboration of the trauma memory into autobiographical memory. Clinical Psychologist Nick Grey (2007) describes the impact of avoidance in a metaphor in which he compares processing the trauma memory to being like it 'going down a conveyer belt' before being stored normally with other memories 'in a filing cabinet'. He contrasts the memories in the filing cabinet as ones which you can control and bring into your awareness at will. With trauma memories, however, this processing into the filing cabinet is blocked, as when the memory comes onto the conveyer belt to be processed, it is pushed off through avoidance strategies. It therefore remains on a loop, returning to the conveyer belt in reliving symptoms such as intrusive memories, before being avoided again.

Following birth, the way in which a trauma memory is 'rehearsed' can influence the way it is constructed into the autobiographical memory base: if negative experiences are reinforced, either through subsequent negative experiences (such as feeding difficulties), or the way in which the birth is – or is not – talked about, a person may become more likely to develop PTSD (Wells, 2000). This was found to be the case for women following childbirth. Briddon et al (2011) demonstrated an association between high levels of memory disorganisation and acute stress symptoms following childbirth at six weeks post-partum. This association was not present at an earlier time-point in the same sample (in the first four days following the birth) suggesting the way in which the memory was processed over the initial postnatal period was linked with the development of symptoms. It is interesting to note that Ayers et al (2016) found that the association between birth factors and PTSD reduces over time, and the associations between PTSD and pre-birth vulnerability and post-partum factors, such as cognitive and coping factors, may increase over time. This finding further reinforces that the birth itself is not the determining factor in whether or not a woman develops PTSD, and there is scope to facilitate or impede her natural recovery in the post-partum period.

The importance of social support

It is also increasingly recognised that adult attachment style is a key process within the development and maintenance of PTSD. In a comprehensive review of trauma-related research, Charuvastra and Cloitre (2008) described the 'social ecology' of PTSD, in which adult attachment and 'social bonds' influence the way in which an individual responds to trauma in a variety of ways. They draw upon a vast body of research showing that a person's perception of their support network before and after a traumatic event is highly associated with their vulnerability to developing PTSD, which they summarise as a 'general and rather robust finding that support helps buffer against psychological distress' (2008, p. 304). This is because social support in general is an effective means of emotional regulation, as seen in the 'affiliative and soothing' system described above. Social support is thought to be so linked to PTSD within the general trauma literature that it has been found to be the second strongest predictor (for example, see Ozer et al, 2003). It appears to be the perceived quality of support (known as 'functional support') rather than the size of the support network (known as 'structural support') that provides the buffering effect. In this way, positive social interactions can provide an internal and external environment which facilitates a person's natural recovery from PTSD, while negative interactions contribute to its maintenance.

When a person is naturally recovering from a trauma, their fearful feelings are gradually decreasing over time, and Charuvastra and Cloitre (2008) describe them as regaining their 'emotional and cognitive equilibrium'. They suggest that social support conveys a message to the traumatised person that they belong to a safe group and that they will be looked after and supported. This finding that social support is associated with PTSD has been found to be true following childbirth. Dekel et al (2017) showed that low levels of social support were found to be associated with the development of PTSD, particularly low family, staff and partner support. Negative social interactions, however, will reinforce feelings of danger and beliefs about the world being hostile. It is interesting to note that positive support is not always associated with a reduction in distress, but unsupportive social responses are strongly associated with psychological distress. This is consistent with the general finding that 'bad is stronger than good' across almost all psychological phenomena (Baumeister et al, 2001). This is thought to have an adaptive function: humans are thought to have heightened attention towards negative stimuli because it signals a need for change and motivates action towards safety.

Charuvastra and Cloitre (2008) argue therefore that social support is an effective emotion regulator, where the behaviour of others can soothe or exacerbate trauma-driven fears. Like Ehlers and Clark (2000), they emphasise the meaning of events as important for how they are experienced. Of particular note within Charuvastra and Cloitre's review is that appraisals of traumatic events that have been caused by humans appear to be particularly fear-inducing. This is why, as mentioned earlier, PTSD following childbirth is, in some crucial ways, distinct from general PTSD populations. A significant risk factor for a woman experiencing birth as traumatic is the behaviour of healthcare staff, particularly when perceived to be dehumanising, disrespectful or uncaring (Elmir et al, 2010). The review by Charuvastra and Cloitre (2008) also examines the importance of 'the first social bond', that is, a person's own attachment in infancy. As we saw in Chapter 1, the attachment relationship between a child and his or her primary caregivers in early life forms a blueprint for how they go on to interact with the world around them. Charuvastra and Cloitre describe emerging evidence from the field of developmental biology which supports this view that the attachment system is called upon throughout a person's life, particularly in times of stress. Within attachment theory, a person who has internalised a secure attachment will instinctively seek safety in important relationships when feeling threatened. People with less secure attachment styles are less likely to have a well-developed social network, and be less able to utilise their social bonds to cope with emotionally distressing events.

The idea that we are hard wired to seek comfort and safety in others was powerfully illustrated back in the 1950s and 1960s in a number of studies by Harry Harlow (for example, see Harlow, 1958). Harlow studied attachment processes by looking at the effects of various social conditions on the later development of infant rhesus monkeys. In one condition, monkeys were isolated from birth for up to one year and then reintroduced to other monkeys. When in isolation, these monkeys engaged in behaviour such as compulsive rocking and clutching their bodies. When reintroduced to other monkeys, they were initially frightened but then became very aggressive in their behaviour towards themselves and others, and unable to communicate with their social group. In another condition, infant monkeys were separated from their birth mother immediately after delivery and placed in a cage with two 'surrogate mothers', one made from wire and the other covered in soft terry towelling cloth. Harlow set this condition up so that four monkeys could obtain milk from the wire 'mother' and four could obtain milk from the cloth 'mother'. It was observed that both groups of monkeys showed a preference for being with the cloth mother. Even those monkeys who obtained milk from the wire mother only went to the wire mother to be fed, and would then return to the comfort of the cloth mother. If a frightening object was placed in the cage, the infant monkeys sought safety with the cloth mother. While the ethics of these studies obviously fall below the rigorous standards we expect today, and are limited by their focus on primates, it is thought that these studies are a compelling demonstration of a natural instinct and need for supportive social interaction and comfort, particularly at times when we are most vulnerable, for example in infancy or in times of trauma and adversity.

More recently, neurobiological studies have shown that early disruptions to attachment can lead to long-term disruptions in the brain's systems for modulating social affiliation, including the ability to be calmed and soothed by social interaction. Charuvastra and Cloitre (2008) explain how early childhood adversity appears to alter these neural systems for social bonding, making it harder for an individual with an insecure attachment to build protective social networks and use their social resources later on when they encounter stress and trauma in their lives. These ideas were further elaborated by Bryant (2016), who described there being overwhelming evidence that social attachments play a critical role in how humans manage adversity. Bryant explains that our ability to engage and co-operate with one another has been central to our survival as a human species, reflected in fundamental neural circuitry that drives our everyday functioning. Bryant also discusses the theory that a person with an anxiously insecure attachment style may be vigilant and detect threat before the securely attached others, and as such act as a 'sentinel' for the wider group. Bryant suggests this may account for up to one third of people having an insecure attachment style: it may heighten individual vulnerability to PTSD but also appears to serve a protective function for the wider social group as a whole. A study by Quinn et al (2015) found that women with an avoidant attachment style were less likely to feel respected by staff during labour, and also more likely to have high levels of hyperarousal in the postnatal period.

While a person with a secure attachment style may feel compelled to seek safety and support from the wider social context following a trauma, it is not always the case that the wider social context is able to provide that support. A woman who has given birth may find themselves cut off from her usual preferred support system for many reasons: being on maternity leave and being isolated from work colleagues and friends, perhaps living away from family and close friends. Her main attachment figure may well be her partner, and if he or she is struggling to come to terms with their own experience of witnessing a traumatic birth, or have a different coping style, this further isolates the traumatised mother. Iles et al (2011) found that less secure attachment and dissatisfaction with partner support were associated with higher levels of both depression and post-traumatic stress in the post-natal period. Evidence also appears to suggest that an insecure attachment will decrease the likelihood of having such a social network of supportive others to turn to. If this is the case for a mother who is feeling traumatised by her birth experience, she starts from a point of isolation without the necessary internal blueprint for how to seek comfort and support in others. Bryant (2016) suggests that people with avoidant attachment tendencies may prefer to engage in other secondary coping strategies to manage their experience, but there has been little research carried out into what these strategies are and whether or not they are adaptive. What is clear, however, is that it is not guaranteed that a woman's natural social group can and will provide the support she as an individual may need following a traumatic birth, and services need to think about a range of ways of helping such women in their recovery.

Charuvastra and Cloitre (2008)'s final 'social bond' under consideration is the one between a traumatised person and their therapist. They describe how a person with PTSD is in a heightened state of fear, with a tendency to perceive threat in the environment: this will include the therapist. They argue that the therapist's first task is to therefore provide the person with a sense of safety through being warm, supportive and interested in the person's experience. It is also important that the therapist seek to understand the meaning of the traumatic experience for the individual. Charuvastra and Cloitre (2008) describe therapy as the creation of a social bond, and the relationship between the person with PTSD and their therapist as a reflection of this bond. We would argue that all healthcare professionals can have the potential to provide women with this healing social bond, as demonstrated by Violet's experience (see Case Study 2.5).

CASE STUDY 2.5 Violet's experience

Violet had her first baby by emergency caesarean section following a long and painful induction at forty-two weeks. When she returned home a couple of days later, she found that she could not stop crying. She felt consumed by wanting to understand why her body had 'failed' – she felt she had failed to go into labour as she should have done, and then she had failed to respond to the induction well enough. She was attempting to breastfeed and finding it an uphill struggle to learn how to latch her baby on without causing her immense pain. Violet felt scared and on edge. Her family and friends came round to meet the baby and Violet felt she must put on a happy face for them, but inside she felt as if she had died: she had a constant feeling of dread and images of the birth kept popping into her mind. She felt that she loved her baby, and certainly did not want to be parted from him, but also felt that maybe she had made a terrible mistake by wanting to have a baby. This thought made her feel completely ashamed; surely she should be over the moon to have a healthy baby? That's what everyone said to her – why couldn't she believe it to be true?

Ten days after the birth, she had a check-up with her community midwife. Violet liked her midwife, she had been very kind during pregnancy and her warm, reassuring manner during check-ups after the baby had been born had helped to put Violet's mind at ease for a short while. During these visits, the midwife had asked Violet how she was feeling, and Violet, fearing she would be judged a bad mother, or a threat to her baby, had said that she felt fine. On day ten, however, Violet felt she could not maintain her happy face any longer and opened up to her midwife about how she had been feeling, sobbing as she did so. The midwife calmly listened, expressed empathy for Violet's distress, and then explained how Violet's feelings were part of her coming to terms with what she had been through. The midwife reassured Violet that she had seen many women feel similar things over the years, but that for most women, these feelings pass – and that help is available for the women where the feelings do not pass. She reassured Violet that it was completely understandable, and not in any way her fault, that she was feeling so overwhelmed. She helped Violet think through where she could get some practical support to allow her to get some rest and gave her some guidance about feeding. Violet left the appointment feeling that the dread had dissipated. Although her mood continued to be up and down for some months after this, when her baby turned one year old, Violet looked back on the time after her baby's birth and how sad and scared she had felt. She had a strong sense that the conversation with her midwife at day ten had been a turning point for her: she had been on track to feeling as if she was sinking further and further into a dark hole with her emotions, but that conversation had reassured her and given her a hope that enabled her to feel less anxious about her emotions, and move forwards in a more positive direction.

The tip of the iceberg?

Building upon the research described above, several frameworks for developing a formulation of PTSD following childbirth have been proposed. Slade (2006) described a two-dimensional model which considered the predisposing, precipitating and maintaining factors involved in a woman's presentation, and how these relate to internal, external and interactional factors. Predisposing factors may relate to a woman's pre-existing personality or attachment style, or her previous history of trauma or mental health difficulties. Precipitating factors refer to those events more directly related to the birth itself, such as obstetric risk factors, while maintaining factors refers to responses and behaviours within the postnatal period which exacerbate symptoms and negative beliefs, or prevent natural recovery from taking place. As described above, these factors intersect with internal, external (or environmental) and interactional factors.

This model is similar to that proposed by Ayers et al (2016), who used the results of a meta-analysis to develop a model of the aetiology of PTSD following childbirth as being the result of the interplay between pre-birth, perinatal and postnatal factors that contribute to presenting difficulties. They build upon the concept of a 'diathesis-stress' model, which proposes that psychological distress is caused by the interaction between predisposing vulnerability factors and the stress caused by specific life experiences. It is the interplay between these different factors which is crucial. For example, trauma history has been found to interact with interventions during the delivery to increase the risk of PTSD, and support during the birth can mediate these pathways (Ford & Ayers, 2011).

When trying to understand how a woman is feeling about her birth experience, it is therefore crucial that we remember that what happened during the birth is only one part of why she is feeling the way she does. How she *felt* about what happened was far more significant. The interaction of a wide range of biological, psychological and social factors have all played a part in her ongoing experience. As trauma responses are so complex, and affected by such a wide range of dynamic influences, it is unhelpful to focus on any one of these areas without considering the others. Vital clues in understanding what has happened, and what is happening now, will be missed if we take a reductionist approach of focusing just on the birth. It is therefore helpful to keep in mind that, although the birth-specific factors are of great importance, they are also the tip of the iceberg in that many other factors are also significant. As discussed in this chapter, there are many other factors which lie beneath the surface, unseen, yet exerting a powerful influence. It is useful to remember this analogy when a woman's emotional reaction and behaviours post-partum seem at odds with our professional interpretation of her birth experience.

The potential for post-traumatic growth

Over recent years, there has been a growing interest in expanding our focus beyond psychopathology and looking as well at beneficial psychological processes. One such process to receive attention has been the area of 'post-traumatic growth'. This can be conceptualised as experiencing positive changes in beliefs or functioning as a result of challenging life events or circumstances (Ayers, 2017). It describes the experience of people who do not just recover from a traumatic event, and return to their pre-trauma functioning, but as a result of their struggle with the trauma, go on to achieve further individual development (Zoellner & Maercker, 2006). This development may take the form of personal benefits, new life priorities, a deepened sense of meaning, or a deepened sense of connection with others or with a higher power. Zoellner and Maercker (2006) explain that post-traumatic growth and PTSD are distinct, independent constructs. Although each construct exists on a continuum, they do not represent opposite ends of the same continuum of adaptation to trauma. Growth and distress may exist simultaneously. Post-traumatic growth, or to use an alternative, but generally synonymous term, 'benefit-finding', has been shown in a meta-analysis to be linked to more intrusive and avoidant thoughts about the trauma, although also related to less depression and more positive affect (Helgeson et al, 2006).

In a parallel with the general trauma literature, Ayers (2017) described how most research into childbirth-related PTSD has focused on risk and distress, but this has overlooked the potentially complementary perspective of investigating positive factors, such as resilience and post-traumatic growth following childbirth. Qualitative research on women's experiences following a traumatic birth experience have found that some women do go on to report positive outcomes such as a sense of strength or purpose (Elmir et al, 2010; Thomson & Downe, 2010). In a prospective, longitudinal design, a sample group of women was assessed for positive change during the third trimester of their pregnancy and again at eight weeks post-partum (Sawyer et al, 2012). Almost half of women reported at least a small degree of positive change following childbirth, measured across five dimensions widely accepted to be associated with the construct of personal growth: 'new possibilities', 'relating to others', 'personal strength', 'spiritual change', and 'appreciation of life' (see the 'Post-Traumatic Growth Inventory' by Tedeschi & Calhoun, 1996). The domain 'appreciation of life' was the most strongly endorsed, with spiritual change the least. Sawyer et al (2012) also found that in general, demographic variables were not related to growth, with only age being significant. In their sample, younger participants reported higher levels of growth, which they speculate may be due to younger women being more open to learning and reappraising their existence. The only birth event variable predictive of growth was type of delivery. Women who had a caesarean section (either elective or emergency) showed higher levels of growth than women having a vaginal delivery, which they hypothesise may relate to the potential for a more stressful experience to stimulate greater growth. Sawyer et al (2012) propose that following childbirth, women may follow the 'curvilinear' relationship between growth and PTSD symptoms identified in the general PTSD literature, in which low levels of distress are not sufficient to induce growth, while overwhelming levels of distress inhibit growth. It is interesting to note that the strongest predictor of growth following childbirth identified by Sawyer et al (2012) was the presence of PTSD symptoms relating to a recent stressful event during pregnancy. Possible explanations for this are that women who are already 'in crisis' have mobilised their coping resources, and prior crisis experience may have enhanced their coping resources further.

Theoretical models seeking to explain post-traumatic growth hypothesise that when a person experiences a trauma, their basic belief system is 'shattered', and they have to then engage in a process of rebuilding their beliefs through cognitive processing and searching for meaning. The outcome of this is that the person feels they have grown through the process (for example, see Janoff-Bulman, 2004). There is some evidence that women engage in this following childbirth as they seek to integrate their memory of the birth. Briddon et al (2015) measured women's emotional experience of birth within three days of delivery, and then measured memories of the birth and emotional adjustment at six weeks post-partum. They found that although the majority of women reported birth as a more negative experience in the immediate days following the delivery, by six weeks, most women reported having only positive memories of it. The degree to which they enjoyed these memories was linked to greater emotional wellbeing in the post-partum. The authors explain this finding in relation to the meta-cognitive model described earlier: the way in which women appraise their memories of a negative event appear to have influenced how the event has become encoded and experienced within memory, and this has been significant for their emotional adjustment. This reflects the dynamic way in which memories are constructed and reconstructed over time, rather than being encoded in a static fashion.

Conclusion

A body of research detailed in this chapter has a consistent finding: it is the woman's subjective experience of the birth that determines whether it activates the 'threat protection system' and is perceived as traumatic. Her pre-existing personality and experiences are also important, as are her coping mechanisms and appraisal of her emotional state afterwards. Social support, from loved ones and professionals, has great power in the post-partum period, to either help to facilitate a woman's natural recovery and 'regain her equilibrium' or exacerbate her distress by confirming and reinforcing her sense of threat and danger.

References

American Psychiatric Association (2013). *Diagnostic and statistical manual of mental disorders* (5th edn). Washington, DC: American Psychiatric Association.

Andersen, L., Melvaer, L., Videbech, P. & Lamont, R. (2012). Risk factors for developing post-traumatic stress disorder following childbirth: a systematic review. *Acta Obstetricia et Gynecologica*, 91, 1261–1272.

Andersen, L., Melvaer, L., Videbech, P., Lamont, R. & Joergensen, J. (2012). Risk factors for developing post-traumatic stress disorder following childbirth: A systematic review. *Acta Obstetrica et Gynecologica Scandinavica*, 91, 1261–1272. doi: 10.1111/j.1600-0412.2012.01476.x.

Ayers, S. (2004). Delivery as a traumatic event: Prevalence, risk factors and treatment for postnatal posttraumatic stress disorder. *Clinical Obstetrics and Gynecology*, 47(3), 552–567.

Ayers, S. (2017). Birth trauma and post-traumatic stress disorder: The importance of risk and resilience. *Journal of Reproductive and Infant Psychology*, 35(5), 427–430.

Ayers, S., Bond, R., Bertullies, S. & Wijma, K. (2016). The aetiology of post-traumatic stress following childbirth: A meta-analysis and theoretical framework. *Psychological Medicine*, 46, 1121–1134.

Ayers, S., Wright, D. & Ford, E. (2015). Hyperarousal symptoms after traumatic and nontraumatic births. *Journal of Reproductive and Infant Psychology*, 33(3), 282–293.

Barclay, L. M. & Lloyd, B. (1996). The misery of motherhood: Alternative approaches to maternal distress. *Midwifery*, 12(3), 136–139.

Bosquet-Enlow, M., Kitts, R., Blood, E., Bizarro, A., Hofmeister, M. & Wright, R. (2011). Maternal posttraumatic stress symptoms and infant emotional reactivity and emotion regulation. *Infant Behaviour and Development*, 34(4). doi: 10.1016/j.infbeh.2011.07.007.

Bennett, H. & Wells, A. (2010). Metacognition, memory disorganisation and rumination in post-traumatic stress symptoms. *Journal of Anxiety Disorders*, 24(3), 318–325.

Brewin, C. (2003). *Posttraumatic stress disorder: Malady or myth?* New Haven, CT: Yale University Press.

Brewin, C., Dalgleish, T. & Joseph, S. (1996). A dual representation theory of posttraumatic stress disorder. *Psychological Review*, 103(4), 670–686.

Brewin, C., Gregory, J., Lipton, M. & Burgess, N. (2010). Intrusive images in psychological disorders: Characteristics, neural mechanisms, and treatment implications. *Psychological Review*, 117, 210–232.

Bateman, L., Jones, C. & Jomeen, J. (2017). A narrative synthesis of women's out-of-body experiences during childbirth. *Journal of Midwifery and Women's Health*, 62(4). doi: 10.1111/jmwh.12655.

Baumeister, R., Bratslavsky, E., Finkenauer, C. & Vohs, K. (2001). Bad is stronger than good. *Review of General Psychology*, 5(4), 323–370.

Briddon, E., Isaac, C. & Slade, P. (2015). The association between involuntary memory and emotional adjustment after childbirth. *British Journal of Health Psychology*, 20(4), 889–903.

Briddon, E., Slade, P., Isaac, C. & Wrench I. (2011). How do memory processes relate to the development of posttraumatic stress symptoms following childbirth? *Journal of Anxiety Disorders*, 25(8), 1001–1007.

Bryant, R. (2016). Social attachments and traumatic stress. *European Journal of Psychotraumatology*, 7. doi:10.3402/ejpt.v7.29065.

Charuvastra, A. & Cloitre, M. (2008). Social bonds and posttraumatic stress disorder. *Annual Review of Psychology*, 59, 301–328.

Czarnocka, J. & Slade, P. (2000). Prevalence and predictors of post-traumatic stress symptoms following childbirth. *British Journal of Clinical Psychology*, 39(1), 35–51.

Dekel, S., Stuebe, C. & Dishy, G. (2017). Childbirth induced posttraumatic stress syndrome: A systematic review of prevalence and risk factors. *Frontiers in Psychology*, 8, 560. doi: 10.3389/fpsyg.2017.00560.

Denkova, E., Dolcos, S. & Dolcos, F. (2012). Reliving emotional personal memories: affective biases linked to personality and sex-related differences. *Emotion*, 12(3), 515–528.

Dikmen-Yildiz, P., Ayers, S. & Phillips, L. (2017). Factors associated with post-traumatic stress symptoms (PTSS) 4–6 weeks and 6 months after birth: A longitudinal population-based study. *Journal of Affective Disorders*, 221, 238–245.

Ehlers, A. & Clark, D. (2000). A cognitive model of posttraumatic stress disorder. *Behaviour Research and Therapy*, 38, 319–345.

Ehlers, A., Hackmann, A. & Michael, T. (2004). Intrusive re-experiencing in post-traumatic stress disorder: Phenomenology, theory and therapy. *Memory*, 12, 403–415.

Elmir, R., Schmied, V., Wilkes, L. & Jackson, D. (2010). Women's perceptions and experiences of a traumatic birth: A meta-ethnography. *Journal of Advanced Nursing*, 66, 2142–2153.

Etheridge, J. & Slade, P. (2017). "Nothing's actually happened to *me*": The experiences of fathers who found childbirth traumatic. *BMC Pregnancy and Childbirth*, 17(80). doi: 10.1186/s12884-017-1259-y.

Fenech, G. & Thomson, G. (2014). 'Tormented by Ghosts of their Past': A meta-synthesis to explore the psychosocial implications of a traumatic birth on maternal wellbeing. *Midwifery*, 30, 185–193.

Ford, E. & Ayers, S. (2011). Support during birth interacts with prior trauma and birth intervention to predict postnatal post-traumatic stress symptoms. *Psychological Health*, 26(12), 1553–1570.

Foy, D. W., Sipprelle, R. C., Rueger, D. B., & Carroll, E. M. (1984). Etiology of posttraumatic stress disorder in Vietnam veterans: analysis of premilitary, military, and combat exposure influences. *Journal of Consulting and Clinical Psychology*, 52(1), 79–87.

Gilbert, P. (2009). Introducing compassion-focused therapy. *Advances in Psychiatric Treatment*, 15(3), 199–208.

Grey, N. (2007). Posttraumatic stress disorder: Treatment. In S. Lindsay & G. Powell (Eds), *The handbook of clinical adult psychology*. London: Routledge.

Harlow, H. (1958). The nature of love. *American Psychologist*, 13, 673–685.

Harris, R. & Ayers, S. (2012). What makes labour and birth traumatic? A survey of intrapartum 'hotspots.' *Psychological Health*, 27(10), 1166–1177.

Helgeson,V., Reynolds, K. & Tomich, P. (2006). A meta-analytic review of benefit finding and growth. *Journal of Consulting and Clinical Psychology*, 74(5), 797–816.

Horsch, A., Brooks, C. & Fletcher, H. (2013). Maternal coping, appraisals and adjustment following diagnosis of fetal anomaly. *Prenatal. Diagnosis*, 33, 1137–1145.

Iles, J., Slade, P. & Spiby, H. (2011). Posttraumatic stress symptoms and postpartum depression in couples after childbirth: The role of partner support and attachment. *Journal of Anxiety Disorders*, 25(4), 520–530.

Janoff-Bulman, R. (2004). Posttraumatic growth: Three explanatory models. *Psychological Inquiry*, 15, 30–34.

Lee, D. (2012). *Recovering from trauma using compassion focused therapy*. London: Robinson.

Loveland Cook, A. C., Flick, H. L., Homan, M. S., Campbell, E. C., McSweeney, E. M. & Gallagher, E. M. (2004). Posttraumatic stress disorder in pregnancy: Prevalence, risk factors, and treatment. *Obstetrics & Gynecology*, 103(4), 710–717. doi:10.1097/01.AOG.0000119222.40241.fb.

McKenzie-Harg, K., Ayers, S., Ford, E., Horsch, A., Jomeen, J., Sawyer, A., Thomson, G. & Slade, P. (2015). Post-traumatic stress disorder following childbirth: An update of current issues and recommendations for future research. *Journal of Infant and Reproductive Psychology*, 33(3), 219–237.

McDonald, S., Slade, P., Spiby, H. & Iles, J. (2011). Post-traumatic stress symptoms, parenting stress and mother-child relationships following childbirth and at 2 years postpartum. *Journal of Psychosomatic Obstetrics and Gynaecology*, 32(3), 141–146.

Olde,E., Kleber, R., van der Hart, O. & Pop, V. (2006). Childbirth and posttraumatic stress responses: A validation study of the Dutch impact of event scale –Revised. *European Journal of Psychological Assessment*, 22(4), 259–267.

Olde, E., van der Hart, O., Kleber, R., van Son, M., Wijnen, H. & Pop, V. (2005). Peritraumatic dissociation and emotions as predictors of PTSD symptoms following childbirth. *Journal of Trauma and Dissociation*, 6(3), 125–142.

Ozer, E., Best, S., Lipsey, T. & Weiss, D. (2003). Predictors of posttraumatic stress disorder and symptoms in adults: A meta-analysis. *Psychological Bulletin*, 129(1), 52–73.

Parfitt, Y., Pike, A. & Ayers, S. (2013). The impact of parents' mental health on parent-baby interaction: A prospective study. *Infant Behaviour and Development*, 36, 599–608.

Quinn, K., Spiby, H. & Slade, P. (2015). A longitudinal study exploring the role of adult attachment in relation to perceptions of pain in labour, childbirth memory and acute traumatic stress responses. *Journal of Infant and Reproductive Psychology*, 33(3), 256–267.

Reynolds, J. L. (1997). Post-traumatic stress disorder after childbirth: The phenomenon of traumatic birth. *Journal of the Canadian Medical Association*, 156, 831–835.

Sawyer, A., Ayers, S., Young, D., Bradley, R. & Smith, H. (2012). Posttraumatic growth after childbirth: A prospective study. *Psychology and Health*, 27, 362–377.

Slade, P. (2006). Towards a conceptual framework for understanding post-traumatic stress symptoms following childbirth and implications for further research. *Journal of Psychosomatic Obstetrics and Gynecology*, 27(2), 99–105.

Thomson, G. & Downe, S. (2010). Changing the future to change the past: Women's experiences of a positive birth following a traumatic birth experience. *Journal of Reproductive and Infant Psychology*, 28(1), 102–112.

Tedeschi, R. & Calhoun, L. (1996). The posttraumatic growth inventory: Measuring the positive legacy of trauma. *Journal of Traumatic Stress*, 9, 455–472.

Wells, A. (2000). *Emotional disorders and metacognition: A practical manual and conceptual guide*. Chichester: Wiley.

Williams, C., Taylor, E. & Schwannauer, M. (2016). A web-based survey of mother-infant bond, attachment experiences, and meta-cognition in posttraumatic stress following childbirth. *Infant Mental Health Journal*, 37(3), 259–273.

Zoellner, T. & Maercker, A. (2006). Posttraumatic growth in clinical psychology – a critical review and introduction of a two component model. *Clinical Psychology Review*, 26(5), 626–653.

3 Communication skills

How to listen

Introduction

Being heard is intrinsically linked to feeling understood, and feeling understood is of key importance for wellbeing (Morelli et al, 2014). In the first two chapters, we have explored the psychological adaptation and impact of childbirth and motherhood. Many women, regardless of whether or not they have experienced birth as traumatic, feel a need to tell their story in order to process it. Many people who undergo a talking therapy comment on how healing it feels just to be listened to. For a person who has experienced a traumatic event, we know that they need to engage in a process of 'autobiographical reasoning' to help them make sense of what has happened and who they are in the face of what they have experienced (Singer & Bluck, 2001). Many other women want to avoid talking about their traumatic birth experiences, but we know from research into PTSD that this actually maintains fear-related symptoms (for example, see Pineles et al, 2011). On a busy postnatal ward, technology and checklists are now the norm, and finding time to listen to women can be difficult; yet effective, timely appropriate communication can make a huge difference to outcomes (Bick, 2010). It is therefore important that we provide women with opportunities to talk about the birth, and when they do so, it is equally important that we listen well. As Carl Rogers asserts (1991): 'Good communication, or free communication, within or between people is always therapeutic' (p. 106).

Person-centred communication: the core conditions

Much of our knowledge and skill in the area of listening comes from the field of person-centred counselling. This is a talking therapy based on creating a setting where the 'client' or 'patient' is able to develop a greater understanding of themselves and think about how to move forwards in their lives. The counsellor achieves this via establishing 'core conditions', which were first set out by the founder of person-centred therapy, Carl Rogers (1961). These conditions are considered to be the foundation of creating a useful experience where a woman who has experienced a traumatic birth can feel heard. Most conversations with women about their birth experience will take place outside of formal counselling, so implementing these conditions within routine appointments, or debriefing sessions can powerfully create the setting for women to experience the healing potential of feeling understood.

Empathy

The first condition is empathy, where the counsellor tries to understand the thoughts and feelings being experienced by the client, sometimes referred to as walking in someone else's shoes. True empathy is distinct from sympathy, which is often thought of as feeling *for* someone. With empathy, the goal is to feel *with* the person. An empathic response acknowledges that the counsellor may not automatically know how the person is feeling, and seeks to understand further the person's internal state. A positive relationship has been found between clinician empathy and better health outcomes, even for physical health conditions such as the management of diabetes (Hojat et al, 2011).

Congruence

Another core condition is thought to be 'congruence', where the counsellor is genuine and authentic in their approach so that the client experiences them as a real person. This allows for the development of a real and trusting relationship in which the client can feel valued. It creates a sense of unease and mistrust for clients when counsellors are not genuine and authentic: if a counsellor is, for example, verbally expressing care and understanding for a client but with a facial expression and body language of disinterest, the client will not feel any trust in the verbal expression. To be congruent, therefore, a counsellor needs to be aware of their own internal experience, and to be able to express this in a way that facilitates the client's own understanding and growth.

Unconditional positive regard

Unconditional positive regard refers to a counsellor's stance in seeing the client as doing the best they can with the resources they have available, even if the client is expressing things that the counsellor finds unpalatable. This does not mean that the counsellor has to agree or collude with everything a client says or does, but holding the principle of unconditional positive regard in mind leads the counsellor to express concern rather than judgement when the client is behaving in an unhelpful way. When a counsellor practises from this position, the client perceives them as warm and accepting, and is therefore able to open up and speak about their thoughts and feelings without fearing criticism or judgement.

According to Rogers, these three conditions make up the foundations of a person-centred intervention. Health services aim to be delivered in a person-centred way (NHSE, 2019), and what that means varies depending on the context. The field of person-centred counselling is built upon the premise that the presence of these three core conditions, *empathy, congruence* and *unconditional positive regard,* can create a setting in which people feel heard, valued, accepted and understood, which then facilitates psychological change and growth. When listening to women after childbirth and helping them to make sense of their experience, it is useful to hold these concepts in mind as a foundation and build the conversation upon them. It is the interplay between these conditions which is considered crucial. Being congruent, and the honesty and transparency which accompanies that, will not be experienced as therapeutic, unless that is held alongside positive regard for the person. Similarly, unconditional positive regard is only useful if communicated via an empathic understanding. Working with these core conditions is complex, and skilled counsellors train for many years to utilise them therapeutically. We can, however, keep them in mind as principles that we try to work consistently with. This may sometimes be challenging, particularly on the occasions where we may find ourselves working with a woman we struggle to empathise with, or feel unconditional positive regard for. Similarly, when we are going through difficulties ourselves and have our own internal emotional state to manage, working in a congruent way may be a struggle. It is normal to find these things challenging, as even very experienced therapists do. The very act of finding them challenging may be telling us that we need to stop and rethink our approach with a woman, a sign that we have not yet established a good rapport, or maybe we are starting to feel burnt-out and in need of some support ourselves. It is only by holding them in mind and trying to practice within their parameters that we can either utilise them to maximise our interactions, or be aware that other issues need to be addressed in order to implement them.

Practical skills

The importance of good communication skills is regularly emphasised in healthcare settings (for example, see Foronda et al, 2016), but too often this focuses on the clinician's ability to articulate clearly, give the right information and ask the right questions. It feels almost counter-intuitive to think about the most important step of communication as being when we are quiet, but as Stickley (2011) explains, listening and non-verbal communication are not passive; they are skills requiring effort and discipline. Communication comprises three elements: the linguistic aspects (the actual words that are articulated), the paralinguistic aspects (how words are articulated, for example, timing, volume, pace) and non-verbal aspects, which relates to body language such as facial expression, bodily position and so on. For communication to be effective there needs to be a two-way process of both articulating clearly, and listening deeply, across all three of these domains. 'Active listening' refers to a set of practical skills that seeks to maximise our ability to really take in what the woman is saying, and for the woman to feel truly heard. It has been shown to be more powerful than giving advice or acknowledging understanding, and communicates that the listener cares about the speaker's thoughts and feelings (Weger et al, 2014). As such, it is widely considered to have 'potential therapeutic value' (Fassaert et al, 2007).

Fassaert et al (2007) explain that active listening has a twofold function. It is a useful communication strategy for recognising and exploring a person's cues, but it also has a non-verbal component which acknowledges the person's suffering and conveys permission for this to be expressed. When listening to a person, how this interaction feels and what the outcome of it is, is multi-faceted. It comprises many factors, including what you say, what you show (your non-verbal communication), what you think, what the person hears, what they notice, what they understand and what they can remember. Using active listening skills can help to utilise these factors in a positive direction.

The OARS model

The OARS model of communication skills grew from a person-centred counselling approach called 'Motivational Interviewing', the origins of which were focused on helping people to make positive changes to their behaviours (Miller & Rollnick, 2002). Motivational Interviewing can be successfully applied by non-mental-health specialists, for example health visitors and midwives (for example, see Chittenden, 2012 and Karatay et al, 2010). The OARS model is therefore a set of skills-based techniques that is accessible and practical to use when having conversations clinically, and especially when talking to women about their childbirth experiences. Consciously applying these skills during clinical interactions will help these conversations be more efficient and effective.

The OARS model covers four basic skills:

- **O**pen questions
- **A**ffirmations
- **R**eflective listening
- **S**ummarising

Open questions

Using open questions, as opposed to closed questions, which usually elicit one-word responses, has a number of functions. Open questions help to explore and gain an understanding of the person's internal and external world, and learn about their experiences, feelings, thoughts, beliefs and behaviours. A useful rule of thumb to indicate whether or not questions are sufficiently open is to gauge who is doing most of the talking during the session: if it is the woman, the questions are probably pitched correctly.

It is worth noting, however, that sometimes, closed questions are appropriate. This is the case when there is a need to clearly understand certain facts or events. It can also be the case when women are particularly anxious and finding it difficult to speak openly; here, the use of a 'reverse funnel', beginning with closed questions and then widening this out into more open questions, can help to establish rapport and facilitate the woman feeling able to speak.

Within the OARS model, it is also recommended to avoid asking 'why' questions; for example, 'why are you no longer breastfeeding?' Questions beginning with 'why' require the person to justify their thoughts or behaviour, and can put them into a defensive position. This then has the potential to negatively impact on rapport and close down a conversation. The OARS model instead suggests reframing questions to begin with 'what' or 'how': 'what factors led you to stop breastfeeding?' or 'how did the decision to stop breastfeeding come about?'

Closed questions are often thought of as those which invite a 'yes/no', or other one-word answer. They can also be stock phrases, which on paper appear to be an open question, but in practice, are well-worn and elicit a standard automatic response. Starting a conversation with 'how are you?' for example, appears to be an open question, but it usually invites the response 'fine, thanks' as this has become another way of greeting a person, rather than a way to open up a genuine conversation. Some clinicians prefer to start the interaction with something that invites less of a socially programmed response, such as 'how have things been going?' or 'what would you like to talk about today?'

Affirmations

A simple affirmation statement to a person about a personal strength, or ability, or positive change they have already made, that you have noticed in them is a very powerful technique that can communicate to a person the value and potential you see in them. It can also build rapport and expand the person's sense of self-efficacy by communicating a belief that they can be responsible for their own positive coping and changes. Verbally this can take the form of statements relating to positive feedback, such as 'it is not always easy to come and talk about the birth again – you showed a lot of courage in coming here today'.

Reflective listening

This is often thought of as the most challenging of the skills within OARS. It requires us to pay close attention to the woman's words and body language, and reflect these using their own words and perceptions. It may be the most challenging skill, but it also has the most potential for creating change in the person's awareness. Using reflective statements demonstrates that you are listening and seeking to understand the person's situation, thoughts and feelings. It also offers the woman the opportunity to hear her own words reflected back to her. Reflections may be offered of a woman's words; for example, 'I heard you say that you felt frightened when the doctor mentioned forceps' or 'you're telling me about how lonely and vulnerable you felt when your partner had to go home'. Reflections may also be offered about a woman's non-verbal communication, including her emotional state (for example, 'you seem to be feeling afraid of being separated from your baby now' or 'I understand why you felt really angry about the way you were spoken to') or behavioural presentation (for example, 'I can see you feel really moved by remembering that aspect of the birth' or 'you smiled when you told me about how good it felt to finally hold your baby').

Summarising

Summarising is also sometimes referred to as paraphrasing. It helps to ensure that the listener and speaker are 'on the same page' during the conversation as it allows the speaker to hear back what the listener has understood. This can either help the speaker to know they have been heard, or gives them the opportunity to correct anything the listener has not understood correctly. When offering a summary, being particularly alert for the woman saying 'yes, but …' is helpful as this is often a sign that she and the listener are not on the same page and that rapport is breaking down. By offering a summary, you are also communicating to the woman that you want to get a full and accurate understanding, which in turn communicates a level of worth and importance to the woman about her feelings and experience. Summaries also help to transition between parts of the conversation and can help to bring the interaction to a close.

The SURETY model

The SURETY model (Stickley, 2011) describes a framework for empathic non-verbal communication to facilitate a practical therapeutic space. Its origins lie within mental health nursing. Stickley (2011) explains that non-verbal communication can create a therapeutic space where the speaker can experience psychological safety and an opportunity to communicate with the listener: 'non-verbal communication is about becoming aware of how we behave in the interpersonal space and deliberatively creating an environment where the space becomes therapeutic and not oppressive' (p. 396).

The SURETY model covers six key concepts:

- **S**it at an angle to the client
- **U**ncross arms and legs
- **R**elax
- **E**ye contact
- **T**ouch
- **Y**our intuition

Sit at an angle to the client

Sitting at a slight angle is thought to create a non-confrontational, comfortable seating arrangement. Strickley (2011) acknowledges that every individual will have their own sense of 'personal space', determined by culture, upbringing and individual preference, and all clues, however small, of discomfort, should be intuitively responded to.

Uncross arms and legs

Crossed arms and legs are thought to signal defensiveness or disinterest. Strickley (2011) argues that deliberately uncrossed arms and legs is a signal to being open and receptive to what the person is saying. Balance is important here, as a slouched position or one that is too open can become a barrier.

Relax

As with the previous point, there is a balance to be struck with this concept, but in essence it relates to feeling relaxed in a comfortable, open posture – but not so relaxed that it signals disinterest. Similarly, Strickley (2011) mentions the need to look 'appropriately concerned' when a person is disclosing disturbing content, but not looking 'over concerned' in an unnatural way.

Eye contact

Appropriate eye contact is a powerful signal of respect and attention, but this is very different to staring, which is experienced as insensitive and intrusive. Similarly, 'wandering eyes', for example, to the clock or other stimuli in the room can be interpreted as a loss of interest. If a time-check is necessary, it is usually better to be explicit about this and state 'I'm just going to check the clock' rather than stealing a furtive glance. Strickley (2011) acknowledges the need for appropriate eye contact to break on occasions, but to have eye contact at the ready if the speaker is looking away. If they look back at the listener and the listener's eyes are not waiting for them, this can be experienced negatively and lead to a loss of rapport.

Touch

Appropriate use of touch is not universal and there can be cultural differences regarding this (Strickley, 2011). Sensitive and respectful use of touch can communicate compassion, empathy and understanding, while inappropriate use of touch can be experienced as abusive. Strickley (2011) refers to body zones which are generally considered 'safe' to potentially touch on adults, when it feels appropriate to do so. He gives the examples of the hand or lower arm, or 'a hand on a shoulder may communicate warmth, care and understanding' (p. 398). Strickley (2011) warns that the therapeutic use of touch is complex and should be guided by good intuitive practice. This is an area that strongly links back to the core conditions described earlier, particularly the need for congruence and being genuine. If touching feels unnatural or uncomfortable, it is better avoided. If there is an intuitive sense that the woman would appreciate the communication of warmth and compassion via touch, and it feels comfortable to do so in an appropriate manner, then it can be a useful tool.

Your intuition

Strickley (2011) explains that while there are no universal guidelines for how a professional may use their intuition in every situation, a clinician will learn to trust their intuition as they grow in professional confidence. He argues that all of the above components of SURETY should be implemented by using intuition, which itself is dependent on individual culture and life experience.

Barriers to communication

Although we know that active listening is important and helpful, it is often harder to do than it sounds. As F. J. Roethlisberger, Professor of Human Relations said, 'When we think about the many barriers to personal communication, particularly those due to differences in background, experience, and motivation, it seems extraordinary that any two people can ever understand each other' (Rogers & Roethlisberger, 1991, p. 108). Given that dissatisfaction with communication is consistently one of the most frequent reasons for complaints within the NHS (Abdelrahman, 2017; NHS Digital, 2018) there are clearly things that get in the way of clinicians being able to communicate in an effective, person-centred way. Being aware of these factors is a useful first step in considering how we may address them at an organisational and individual level. Within healthcare settings, it is useful to consider these barriers within three domains: clinician factors, patient factors, and institutional factors (Granek et al, 2013).

Clinician factors

When being trained in communication skills, a commonly held fear by health professionals who are not specialists in mental health is the idea that if they facilitate a person talking about their feelings, they will be 'opening up a can of worms', which they then do not have the time to explore, or know how to safely close. For many clinicians, a lack of time is the most immediate barrier to feeling able to engage in conversations with women about their birth experience in depth and with a focus on the emotional aspects of the experience. Many clinicians work in settings where they are carrying out busy clinics or working in hectic ward environments. Clinicians sometimes report that within their role, they have a specific set of things that 'must be done' with a woman; for example a health visitor carrying out a two-week check often has a packed agenda of things to cover in that visit, with many more visits waiting for them that day. It can be challenging, in these kinds of circumstances, to spend time with a woman you suspect may be struggling, gently exploring her feelings, when the reality is that there is not the time to do so in depth. It is not ideal, but a compromise in these situations is to communicate to the woman that how she is feeling is very important, and you would like to have the opportunity to talk with her about it in more detail when there is time to do so properly. In these circumstances, you can then arrange a time and resume the conversation then. Sometimes, we get the sense when talking to a woman that we are seeing a window of opportunity with them to have a conversation about their feelings, and if it is not taken then, it may not present again. This is a difficult decision to make when there are many competing demands for time and attention. It is sometimes useful to remember that a warm, empathic and understanding conversation with good active listening skills is an investment that may save time later on, for yourself or for the wider health system, depending on your role.

Another barrier that can make it feel challenging to 'open the can of worms' is if we do not feel appropriately skilled to have conversations with women who may be in distress or presenting with symptoms of mental health problems. Again, it is a good investment of time to undertake training and seek support in having these conversations. One in four people in the general population will experience a mental health problem (McManus et al, 2009), and 13 per cent of women experience mental health problems postnatally (World Health Organization, 2008). If your role involves working with women in the postnatal period it is therefore likely that a significant number of these will be experiencing some degree of emotional distress. Feeling confident and supported to be able to listen to their feelings and experiences is an essential skill to have. Employers should also recognise this and provide training in communication skills, as well as ongoing support and supervision.

Even the most skilled and experienced clinician, who generally feels very confident in their communication skills, may find this ability tested from time to time. This may happen in relation to certain people, for example, women who we just find it difficult to make a connection with. It may also relate to times where we are experiencing struggles in our own lives which may leave us feeling too 'full' of our own emotion to be able to focus on the woman's. Some psychotherapists refer to the concept of 'containment', an idea dating back to one of the prominent figures in our modern understanding of psychotherapy, Walter Bion (1962). Bion's theory of containment drew from the observation that in normal development, a baby projects his or her upsetting and unbearable feelings onto the mother. Because of the strong link between the mother and baby, the mother is able to feel the baby's emotion, take it in and contain it, giving it back to the baby in a safer, more bearable form. This concept has since been applied to the therapeutic process, in which the therapist provides a safe space which can contain the emotions of the client, allowing them to observe and process feelings they would otherwise find overwhelming and unbearable. It is not unique to the mother–baby or therapist–client relationships; all emotionally supportive relationships in which one person seeks to understand and care for the feelings of another includes an element of containment. It is why we say, 'a problem shared is a problem halved', because the distress is being at least partly contained by another person. Containment is also happening when women are discussing their disturbing feelings relating to their birth experience: they are using us as a container for their distress so that they can process and make sense of it. When we as clinicians find ourselves unable to provide this containing space, it is often because we are full of our own emotional state, sometimes associated with work-related issues, and sometimes associated with our personal lives. Sometimes, our feelings may be very specific to the nature of the conversation at hand; it may be the case that particular aspects of a woman's experience resonate with your own, and this triggers a personal emotional response. Talking to women about birth can be potentially very evocative, triggering us to remember and reflect on our own reproductive histories and experiences. It is why access to restorative supervision and self-reflection are crucial aspects of professional practice when doing emotional work. This is explored in more depth in Chapter 7.

Carl Rogers (in Rogers & Roethlisberger, 1991) described 'the tendency to evaluate', by which he meant the natural urge to judge and approve or disapprove of the other person's statement. He argued that this impulse to evaluate any emotionally meaningful statement from our own viewpoint blocks interpersonal communication. Rogers (1991) suggested that we overcome this when we listen with real understanding, seeing the expressed idea from the other person's point of view, sensing how it feels to them and achieving their frame of reference about the subject under discussion. He explains that we find it difficult to listen with understanding because it involves taking a risk: he describes that entering another person's internal world and seeing the way life appears to them, has the potential for you to also be changed yourself in that you might come to see things the way the person does, or your own attitudes or personality may be changed.

Working emotionally requires a significant paradigm shift for clinicians who have trained either in a medical model, or whose training is focused primarily on delivering physical care. This training can programme us into wanting to focus on the physical aspects of a person's presentation at the expense of their psychological state: we may be more prone to doing this when we feel overwhelmed or unskilled to work in a psychological way. Within the Motivational Interviewing approach described earlier, Miller and Rollnick (2004) explain how clinicians can feel an urge to provide advice or reassurance, which they call 'the righting reflex'. Unfortunately, they also explain how research has consistently shown that the more we tell people what to do, the less likely they are to actually do it, so the righting reflex is often unsuccessful. It can also feel uncomfortable to allow a woman to become distressed without offering immediate comfort and reassurance. Again, the urge to do so can feel like an automatic reflex response in people who have trained to be healthcare professionals out of a desire to alleviate distress and provide comfort. The difficulty is that offering comfort and reassurance too soon can be experienced as closing down a conversation. Safely containing a woman's distress while she opens up about her experience and feelings allows for a full exploration of her internal state, and facilitates an in-depth understanding.

Patient factors

There may also be aspects of a woman's presentation that make it difficult for her to engage in a conversation about her experience and feelings. Her emotional state may be such that it makes communication challenging. Severe depression can affect a person's cognitive functioning such that they may struggle to think clearly, concentrate and articulate themselves (for example, see Austin et al, 2001 and Castaneda et al, 2008). Her prior mental health and birth experience will also influence how she approaches the conversation. Some women may be highly sensitive to shame in such interactions (Gilbert, 2000) and if already feeling high levels of shame, the communication of the clinician will be interpreted through this lens. She may then, for example, perceive the clinician's neutral words as critical. This is particularly important when a woman has experienced her care as inadequate during the birth: she may be entering the conversation with a belief that clinicians are not to be trusted and will let her down. She may also feel trepidation that the healthcare system will 'close ranks' and be defensive about any shortcomings, rather than being open and willing to listen. This will again affect her own communication style, either making her feel defensive and hostile or particularly vulnerable and unsafe. Being well equipped in communication skills will help clinicians to navigate these challenging conversations, being mindful of how the woman is experiencing them.

Some women have existing neurodevelopmental conditions that may affect their communication style, such as autistic spectrum conditions. It may be that this is known prior to the conversation, but it is also important to be conscious that conditions such as autism are under-recognised in women, and it is therefore likely that some women may present to services without knowing themselves that they would meet criteria for an autistic spectrum condition. It is worth considering this as a possibility when listening to a woman who appears to be struggling with the social interaction and communication aspect of having a conversation about their birth experience. This is particularly important as research has shown that non-autistic individuals form less favourable first impressions of people with autism, and are less willing to interact with them face-to-face (Sasson et al, 2017). So that women with autism are not prevented from accessing helpful conversations to aid them in their processing of their birth experience, we should be alert to the possibility of undiagnosed autism being present, and able to modify our communication style accordingly. It is recommended that we allow women time to process what has been said, avoid the use of too many questions and minimise interference from any environmental sensory distractions. Similarly, be aware that some women may have a more concrete thinking style and therefore find it difficult to understand and connect with the use of metaphor. I once, for example, used the phrase 'dip your toe in' to a woman and rather than convey a sense of trying something out without becoming fully committed, the woman went on to tell me about her feelings about swimming. It can also be helpful to bear in mind that non-verbal communication may be different too; some women with autism may, for example, have a different use of eye contact. Some women may find eye contact too intense and look away when thinking or answering questions. This can be a sign that they are trying very hard to participate in the conversation, rather than being a sign of disengagement. As with all communication principles, it is important to apply them with flexibility and understand that all communications may have individualised meanings dependent on the woman, whatever her neurodevelopmental status.

Most of the evidence about effective communication has come from the fields of counselling and psychotherapy, a model which is traditionally most often delivered in a one-to-one format. In practice, this will not always be the case when talking to women about their birth experience. She may have her baby, or other children present. The impact of this can be twofold: we have a duty of care to the baby or children, to protect them from the potential disturbance they may feel if they witness their mother becoming too upset, and the presence of children may be a distraction for the woman that prevents her from focusing on the conversation. It would be unrealistic and prohibitive to expect women to only ever talk about their birth experience without their baby or other children present, so we must be mindful of the impact the presence of the woman's dependents in the room may be having.

As well as having children present, some women may also have their partner or other family members or friends with them when talking about the birth. We need to be aware of how the presence of others may be facilitating her feeling safe to speak, or inhibiting her. There may be scenarios that are obviously concerning, such as when a partner is present and the clinician picks up on cues that are suggestive of domestic violence and the need for safeguarding. Other scenarios are less obvious but may still need consideration. A woman may have her own mother or caring other present for example, who offers the woman well-meaning comfort if she becomes distressed, such as, 'there, there, now don't get upset, have a tissue and don't cry'. This may be in direct contrast to the stance the clinician is trying to take in allowing the woman to feel emotional, but can also provide the clinician with useful information for understanding how able the woman is to openly discuss and process the birth with her natural support network. Where it is felt that the presence of other people may be inhibiting a woman from being able to openly express her thoughts and feelings, you may find it useful to consider arranging to see the woman separately on a one-to-one basis.

Institutional and social factors

Relating to the fears some clinicians express in their reluctance to 'open a can of worms' is a concern that if they do discuss a woman's feelings and find that she is symptomatic of PTSD or other significant mental health problem, there may not be the pathways in place to refer her on for further support. As outlined in Chapter 5, some areas do have access to specialist psychological support, but even where this is available, it is often a very limited resource. All women, however, can access psychological support via their GP or self-referral into local Improving Access to Psychological Therapies (IAPT) services. While this route does lack the specialist knowledge and close links with midwifery and obstetric services that can enhance a woman's psychological care, generic IAPT services should have provision to treat PTSD in accordance with NICE guidelines (NICE, 2018).

Although it is thankfully an improving landscape, talking about mental health can still carry significant stigma and this can also prevent women from talking about their experiences and subsequent difficulties. This can be particularly problematic in the field of maternal mental health as it can still feel 'taboo' to talk about having experienced birth as traumatic. Our clinical experience is that women have often been reluctant to seek help because they feel society expects them to feel lucky to have had a baby, and that they are somehow a weak or inadequate mother for having any negative feelings. There can also be a fear for some women that if she admits to professionals that she is struggling with her mental health, they will assume she cannot care for her baby and Social Services will become involved. It is therefore important that maternity care is psychologically informed at all levels of the service, for psychological distress to be normalised and wellbeing prioritised, so that women are given the message that their mental health matters throughout their maternity care. Alongside the work of third party organisations to raise awareness of maternal mental health and the ambitions laid out in the NHS Long-term Plan (2019) prioritising mental health and giving women permission to safely express their experiences will allow for more open and honest, and ultimately helpful communication to take place.

Cultural considerations

Healthcare is now provided in a multicultural, multi-ethnic and multiple language society, and yet the cultural context of healthcare, specifically midwifery, has not been well researched, according to Meddings and Haith-Cooper (2008). They point out that childbirth is a time when cultural traditions become more salient, and a midwife must therefore endeavour to develop an understanding of women's cultural perspectives because this may impact on how the woman makes choices. They cite the example of how Western views of autonomy may differ according to different cultural contexts, with some more traditional societies tending to adopt a paternalistic approach to healthcare, with some women doubting their own ability to make choices, deferring instead to the professionals.

There can be challenges associated with providing care to people from different ethnic and cultural backgrounds, which is particularly heightened when people speak little or limited English. Every language has nuances of meaning which configure the language of subjective experience and emotion (Leanza et al, 2014). When healthcare professionals are unable to communicate effectively, they may become angry and frustrated, which the patient may become aware of via non-verbal cues, making them in turn feel vulnerable and inadequate (Meddings & Haith-Cooper, 2008). There are further challenges even when people from different cultures have good language competence: different cultures carry specific terminology, meanings and metaphors that can be hard to navigate (Meuter et al, 2015). As Tribe and Morrissey (2004) point out, languages are not interchangeable. They advise against using metaphors, for example, because of the potential for misunderstandings as these are so culturally embedded. Some emotions with a precise name in one language are not easily translatable, and translating emotional meaning often involves also understanding social contexts and wider culture (Leanza et al, 2014).

Regarding the use of interpreters, Meddings and Haith-Cooper (2008) recommend the use of a tiered structure of language support, acknowledging that the need for communication is on a continuum. They suggest that staff with basic language skills could facilitate social engagement within maternity care, with professional interpreters utilised to transfer the most vital information. Because language is 'the central vehicle' in mental healthcare (Leanza et al, 2014), the use of interpreters is highly recommended when talking to women who have limited English about their childbirth experiences. Some people may feel uncomfortable with an interpreter being present, however, due to concerns about confidentiality or shame (Tribe & Morrissey, 2004). Thorough explanations about the interpreter's code of ethics, and contract around confidentiality will be useful. The use of family members as interpreters is discouraged where possible (Tribe & Morrissey, 2004) because of the potential for negative consequences on the person and family member, and lack of appropriate training. Where conversations about the birth occur unexpectedly in the context of routine care, with a family member acting as interpreter, it would be consistent with Leanza et al's (2014) guidance to roughly evaluate the nature of the problem and then inform the woman of the need to continue the conversation in another session, with the help of a professional interpreter in order to protect all family members and allow the woman to speak as openly as she wishes to. Leanza et al (2014) call for the clinician and professional interpreter to develop a collaborative relationship, where the interpreter can enact a dual role of 'culture broker', explaining differences in values and practices as well as translating language. There are many different issues to consider when working with interpreters, for example, whether their gender will have an impact on a woman's openness to communicate, or the possibility they may be vicariously traumatised by hearing a woman's trauma-related narrative (Leanza et al, 2014).

Clinicians should explore the meanings of cultural differences and similarities rather than assume that all people will have a similar perspective based on their gender, ethnicity or race (La Roche & Maxie, 2003). This may require clinicians to examine their own feelings arising from working within cultural diversity; supervision can be a good forum for this reflection. In general, approaching conversations about women's experience of birth in a curious, non-judgemental stance is useful in facilitating a good understanding within a cross-cultural context.

Useful things to listen for

When communicating with women about their childbirth experiences, there are several features that may be useful to listen for. These features may be indicators of how the woman's experience is affecting her psychologically, and what may be helpful. Symptoms of PTSD and PND are covered in Chapter 2, and of course, it is important to 'have your radar up' to listen out for these (see also Chapter 4). Where there is concern that women may be presenting with clinically significant symptoms, onward referrals for further assessment and support are often indicated (as discussed in Chapter 5). For all women, however, having your radar up for the features described below can often help to guide conversations and provide the woman with useful insights.

Risk

It is well established that suicide is a leading cause of maternal mortality (Knight et al, 2017). It is therefore important to listen out for signs that women may be experiencing suicidal ideation or thoughts of self-harm when talking about their psychological distress during the postnatal period. Signs that someone may be at risk include describing feelings of hopelessness and worthlessness, or feeling as if their family and baby would be better off without them. If you are concerned that someone is feeling suicidal, it is crucial to gather more information about what thoughts they are having, and how significant these thoughts are. Some people who are very psychologically distressed may experience a degree of fantasising that they may be better off dead, which can reflect a wish to escape from what feels like a desperate situation. For many people, their thoughts do not go beyond this level of fantasy, but for some, they do then go on to think about how they may end their life, and begin to make plans. It is therefore imperative to assess not just the thoughts that a person is having, but also whether they are making any plans, and if they have the means and intent to implement those plans. It is also important to ask people about their protective factors to determine what may be the things that stop them from wanting to act on their thoughts. Asking people about any previous experience of suicide or self-harm is also important information. Once you have gathered this information, you can advise the person to seek immediate help (for example, through the Samaritans or local A&E departments), or contact their mental health team if they are under the care of one. For midwives and health visitors vising women post-partum there will be an established route to access perinatal mental health services including out of hours services. If you do not deem the person to be at immediate risk of harm, contact their GP, or, where applicable, their health visitor, to pass on your concerns. Some women may not want you to pass this information on, but concerns about risk usually outweigh confidentiality, and this is why many counselling conversations begin with an explanation that confidentiality is a limited principle, and will be overruled when there are concerns about safety. Having this conversation before a woman begins to tell you about her own feelings means she is fully aware of the consequences if she discloses any suicidal or other concerning information.

It can be very anxiety-provoking to talk to someone who is considering suicide. Being able to discuss these conversations with colleagues and share any concerns is therefore crucial in order for the best possible decisions to be made, and for the health professional in question to also feel supported. It is important to know your local procedures and systems for managing risk.

Shame

Shame has been described as a 'toxic cocktail' of emotions (Lee, 2012). It is thought to involve two key components: how we feel we exist in the minds of others, and how we evaluate ourselves, a major feature of which is self-criticism (Gilbert & Procter, 2006). Shame is associated with the development of both depression and PTSD (Hoffart et al, 2015; Priel & Besser, 1999). In new mothers experiencing emotional distress, feelings of shame can prevent them from seeking help (Dunford & Granger, 2017) so it is especially important to listen out for signs that a woman may be feeling this way in order to address this. Deborah Lee (2012) explains that experiencing a traumatic event can lead to people feeling ashamed about who they are and what they have been through, as well as feeling ashamed of how they are coping. This feels particularly salient for women who have experienced a traumatic birth as they have absorbed the many unhelpful messages within society about what a good birth *should* be like, and how a good mother *should* behave. Feeling that they are not 'measuring up' to these supposed cultural ideals can lead some women to become highly self-critical and as a result, feel ashamed. Often these thoughts are so automatic the woman is not aware of her response, helping to identify this can be a useful step for women to realise how harshly they are relating to themselves and begin to develop more self-compassion. Listening with care and compassion to women who feel this sense of shame is enormously powerful:

> Shame hates it when we reach out and tell our story. It hates having words wrapped around it – it can't survive being shared … Trust me when I tell you that shame and fear can't tolerate that kind of powerful connection surging between people.
>
> (Brown, 2010, pp. 10–11)

Strengths

Promoting empowerment by focusing on coping is one of the key skills highlighted in Lundeby et al's (2015) model for responding to patients in emotional distress. By focusing on a person's strengths and resources we can learn about their previous coping strategies, potentially increase awareness of their current coping behaviour, overcome barriers for change and empower the patient to utilise and improve their current coping strategies (Stensrud et al, 2014). Listening out for strengths is therefore another useful tool that can stimulate emotional recovery and change.

Conclusion

As healthcare professionals, communication is a vital and inherent part of our job, and the nuance and skill of effective communication need to be continually practised, adapted and honed. We may not always get it right, but we should never underestimate just how therapeutic a person-centred approach to communication can be for women in the post-partum, especially the act of listening.

References

Abdelrahman, W. & Abdelmageed, A. (2017). Understanding patient complaints. BMJ, 356, j:452. doi: https://doi.org/ 10.1136/bmj.j452.

Austin, M., Mitchell, P. & Goodwin, G. (2001). Cognitive deficits in depression: possible implications for functional neuropathology. *British Journal of Psychiatry*, 178, 200–206.

Bick, D. (2010). Communication, communication, communication. *Midwifery*, 26, 377–378.

Bion, W. (1962). Attacks on linking. In E. Bott Spillius (ed.), *Melanie Klein today: Developments in theory and practice*, Vol. 1: *Mainly theory*. London: Routledge.

Brown, B. (2010). *The gifts of imperfection*. Center City, MN: Hazelden.

Castaneda, A., Tuulio-Henriksson, A., Marttunen, M., Suvusaari, J. & Lonnqvist, J. (2008). A review on cognitive impairments in depressive and anxiety disorders with a focus on young adults. *Journal of Affective Disorders*, 106(1–2), 1–27.

Chittenden, D. (2012). A concept analysis of motivational interviewing for the community practitioner. *Community Practice*, 85(10), 20–23.

Dunford, E. & Granger, C. (2017). Maternal guilt and shame: Relationship to postnatal depression and attitudes towards help-seeking. *Journal of Child and Family Studies*, 26(6), 1692–1701.

Fassaert, T., van Dulmen, S., Schellevis, F. & Bensing, J. (2007). Active listening in medical consultations: Development of the Active Listening Observation Scale (ALOS-global). *Patient Education and Counselling*, 68, 258–264.

Foronda, C., MacWilliams, B. & McArthur, E. (2016). Interprofessional communication in healthcare: An integrative review. *Nurse Education in Practice*, 19, 36–40.

Gilbert, P. (2000). The relationship of shame, social anxiety and depression: The role of the evaluation of social rank. *Clinical Psychology and Psychotherapy*, 7(3). doi: 10.1002/1099-0879(200007)7:3<174::AID-CPP236>3.0.CO;2-U.

Gilbert, P. & Procter, S. (2006). Compassionate mind training for people with high shame and self-criticism: Overview and pilot study of a group therapy approach. *Clinical Psychology and Psychotherapy*, 13, 353–379.

Granek, L., Krzyzanowska, M., Tozer, R. & Mazzota, P. (2013). Oncologists' strategies and barriers to effective communication about the end of life. *Journal of Oncology Practice,* 9(4), 129–135.

Hoffart, A., Oktedalen, T. & Langkaas, T. (2015). Self-compassion influences PTSD symptoms in the process of change in trauma-focused cognitive behavioural therapies: A study of within-person processes. *Frontiers in Psychology*, 6. doi: 10.3389/fpsyg.2015.01273.

Hojat, M., Louis, D., Markham, F., Wender, R., Rabinowitz, C. & Gonnella, J. (2011). Physicians' empathy and clinical outcomes for diabetic patients. *Academic Medicine*, 86(3), 359–364.

Karatay, G., Kublay, G. & Emiroglu, O. (2010). Effect of motivational interviewing on smoking cessation in pregnant women. *Journal of Advanced Nursing*, 66(6), 1328–1337.

Knight, M., Nair, M., Tuffnell, D., Shakespeare, J., Kenyon, S., Kurinczuk, J. J. (eds) [on behalf of MBRRACE-UK]. (2017). *Saving lives, improving mothers' care – Lessons learned to inform maternity care from the UK and Ireland Confidential Enquiries into Maternal Deaths and Morbidity 2013–15.* Oxford: National Perinatal Epidemiology Unit, University of Oxford.

La Roche, M. & Maxie, A. (2003). Ten considerations in addressing cultural differences in psychotherapy. *Professional Psychology: Research and Practice*, 34(2), 180–186.

Leanza, Y., Miklavcic, A., Boivin, I. & Rosenberg, E. (2014). Working with interpreters. In L. J. Kirmayer, J. Gudzer & C. Rosseau (eds), *Cultural consultation: Encountering the other in mental health care, international and cultural psychology*. New York: Springer Science and Business Media.

Lee, D. (2012). *Recovering from trauma using compassion focused therapy*. London: Robinson.

Lundeby, T., Gulbrandsen, P. & Finset, A. (2015). The Expanded Four Habits Model – A teachable consultation model for encounters with patients in emotional distress. *Patient Education and Counselling*, 98, 598–603.

McManus, S., Meltzer, H., Brugha, T., Bebbington, P. & Jenkins, R. (2009). *Adult psychiatric morbidity in England, 2007: Results of a household survey.* London: The National Centre for Social Research.

Meddings, F. & Haith-Cooper, M. (2008). Culture and communication in ethically appropriate care. *Nursing Ethics*, 15(1), 52–61.

Meuter, R., Gallois, C., Segalowitz, N., Ryder, A. & Hocking, J. (2015). Overcoming language barriers in healthcare: A protocol for investigating safe and effective communication when patients or clinicians use a second language. *BMC Health Services Research*, 15(371). doi: 10.1186/s12913-015-1024-8.

Miller, W. R. & Rollnick, S. (2002). *Motivational interviewing: Preparing people for change* (2nd edn). New York: Guildford Press.

Miller, W. & Rollnick, S. (2004). Talking oneself into change: Motivational interviewing, stages of change, and therapeutic process. *Journal of Cognitive Psychotherapy*, 18(4), 299–308.

Morelli, S., Torre, J. & Eisenberger, N. (2014). The neural bases of feeling understood and not understood. *Social, Cognitive and Affective Neuroscience*, 9(12), 1890–1896.

NHS Digital (2018). *Data on written complaints in the NHS, 2017–2018.* Available online: https://digital.nhs.uk/data-and-information/publications/statistical/data-on-written-complaints-in-the-nhs/2017–18 [Accessed 4 August 2019].

NHSE (2019). *The NHS Long Term Plan.* Available online: www.longtermplan.nhs.uk/wp-content/uploads/2019/01/nhs-long-term-plan-june-2019.pdf [Accessed 4 August 2019].

NICE [National Institute for Health and Clinical Excellence] (2018). *Post traumatic stress disorder: Management*. NICE guideline (CG116).

Pineles, S., Mostoufi, S., Ready, C., Street, A., Griffin, M. & Resick, P. (2011). Trauma reactivity, avoidant coping, and PTSD symptoms: A moderating relationship? *Journal of Abnormal Psychology*, 120(1), 240–246.
Priel, B. & Besser, A. (1999). Vulnerability to postpartum depressive symptomatology: Dependency, self-critcism and the moderating role of antenatal attachment. *Journal of Social and Clinical Psychology*, 18(2), 240–253.
Rogers, C. (1961). *On becoming a person: A therapist's view of psychotherapy*. London: Constable.
Rogers, C. & Roethlisberger, F. J. (1991). Barriers and gateways to communication. *Harvard Business Review*, Nov–Dec, 105–111.
Sasson, N., Faso, D., Nugent, J., Lovell, S., Kennedy, D. & Grossman, R. (2017). Neurotypical peers are less willing to interact with those with autism based on thin slice judgements. *Scientific Reports*, 7. doi: 10.1038/srep40700.
Singer, J. & Bluck, S. (2001). New perspectives on autobiographical memory: The integration of narrative processing and autobiographical reasoning. *Review of General Psychology*, 5(2), 91–99.
Stensrud, T., Gulbrandsen, P., Mjaaland, T., Skretting, S. & Finset, A. (2014). Improving communication in general practice when mental health issues appear: Piloting a set of six evidence-based skills. *Patient Education and Counselling*, 95, 69–75.
Stickley, T. (2011). From SOLER to SURETY for effective non-verbal communication. *Nurse Education in Practice*, 11, 395–398.
Tribe, R. & Morrissey, J. (2004). Good practice issues in working with interpreters in mental health. *Intervention,* 2(2), 129–142.
Weger, H., Castle Bell, G., Minei, E. & Robinson, M. (2014). The relative effectiveness of active listening in initial interactions. *International Journal of Listening*, 28(1), 13–31.
World Health Organization (2008). *The World Health Report 2008: Primary health care (now more than ever)*. Geneva: World Health Organization.

4 Birth afterthoughts

A stepped care model

Introduction

As discussed in the preceding chapters, women often feel a need to talk through their birth experience in the days and weeks after birth, yet creating the conditions and finding the time to listen can be challenging for busy clinicians. In addition, there continues to be confusion around services which are aimed at providing this type of service to women post-partum and whether they should be routinely offered to women at all. This is in part due to the problem with the term *debriefing* which is so often attached to such services. The term *debriefing* is often used interchangeably and without consensus around its actual meaning (Baxter et al, 2014). In post-partum services it is often used to describe an informal exchange of information allowing the mother to talk about her birth experience and for the midwife to help her make sense of events (Ayers et al, 2006) and whilst women value these opportunities to talk about their birth experience (Borg Cunen et al, 2014; Small et al, 2000), it is not the same as structured *debriefing*. Similarly the Royal College of Obstetricians and Gynaecologists (RCOG) recommends that obstetricians *review* patients prior to discharge to explain the reason for intervention, implications, complications and impact on future deliveries (RCOG, 2011). This type of review is written in medical notes and frequently referred to by clinicians as a 'debrief' (Touqmatchi et al, 2011).

Psychological debriefing

Psychological debriefing is a systematic process which aims to modify thought processes, feelings and memories elicited following a traumatic or stressful event; it allows emotional release and enables cognitive reorganisation (Fullerton et al, 2000). Within healthcare, psychological debriefing has its roots in emergency care with the use of critical incident stress (CIS) debriefing aimed at reducing psychological distress in both patients and staff (Rose et al, 2002). CIS debriefing is used with groups of people who have all been exposed to the same event or type of event, this enables commonality of feelings and reactions to be normalised through sharing and enabling of social support. Group sessions and/or single session debriefing has been used following natural disasters and terrorist attacks (Brewin et al, 2008), and has also been adopted by the military to support military personnel following traumatic events (Greenberg et al, 2010). The overarching principle is to assist coping and reduce further distress and ultimately prevent PTSD occurring after a traumatic event (Rose et al, 2002). When considering its use in the post-partum period it is important to note that this type of post-trauma debriefing is intended to be used within the first few days following an event (Dyregov, 1989) or at least within the first month (Rose et al, 2002) and is usually offered universally to those involved in a trauma as a means of preventing longer-term psychological morbidity. This one size fits all approach highlighted the problem of identifying those at risk of PTSD longer term, for as discussed in Chapter 2 PTSD is not normally diagnosed until at least six weeks post-partum. What is perceived as traumatic to one person is not always perceived as traumatic by all. Additionally as discussed in Chapter 2, acute stress reactions post-trauma will usually reduce and/or disappear over time and can be considered part of the normal neurobiological and cognitive processing of an event. In one study exploring PTSD rates amongst non-sexual assault victims, 70 per cent of women were diagnosed with PTSD symptoms at nineteen days but at a four-month follow-up this had dropped to 21 per cent. In the male sample the rates changed from 50 per cent to zero (Riggs et al, 1995). Offering early (within the first few days or weeks) psychological interventions such as debriefing to all those involved in a trauma-related event with the aim of reducing the incidence of PTSD is not now recommended and in addition may cause more harm than good in certain individuals by interfering with their natural recovery process (Roberts et al, 2009; Rose et al, 2002). This suggests that debriefing should only be offered selectively to those who would not be likely to recover naturally, but currently, no widely used clinical tools are available to accurately predict who is likely to develop PTSD and who is not, because of the wide variety and complexity of predictive variables. Research is continuing with the aim of finding a predictive model which calculates and quantifies individual risk of developing psychological morbidity. One such study (Shalev et al, 2019) has had some success assessing the variables of gender, ethnicity, educational attainment, lifetime history of trauma exposure, and current trauma type, considered as additional predictors of PTSD which could be used in a predictive model.

Understanding the evidence: to debrief or not to debrief post-partum

Until the publication of the first Cochrane Systematic Review on the efficacy of debriefing (Rose et al, 2002) postnatal debriefing services had been recommended as part of routine maternity care by the Audit Commission (1997) with the aim of improving women's experience of maternity care, albeit with no supporting definition or evidence of benefit post-partum. The Cochrane Systematic Review (Rose et al, 2002) included fifteen studies with populations including soldiers, trauma patients and relatives of trauma victims. Three studies were based on an obstetric population (Lavender & Walkinshaw, 1998; Priest et al, 2003; Small et al, 2000). The review concluded that compulsory debriefing of victims of trauma should cease, following this the National Institute for Health and Care Excellence (NICE) (NICE, 2007) recommended that postnatal debriefing should not routinely form part of postnatal care.

Many maternity units still continue to offer services such as *birth afterthoughts* or *birth reflections* which are often badged as 'debriefing services' (Thomson & Garrett, 2019), whereby women can talk about their birth experience and have aspects and outcomes explained, usually by a midwife. In response the research community has continued to explore the relationship between a potentially traumatic event (birth), postnatal debriefing (intervention) and impact on psychological morbidity (Meades et al, 2011). This has been done primarily with targeting women considered 'at risk' of a traumatic birth including instrumental delivery (Kershaw et al, 2005; Small et al, 2000) and emergency caesarean section (Ryding et al, 2004) with no demonstrable effect on rates of PTSD or depressive symptoms. More recently a Cochrane Systematic review (Bastos et al, 2015) concluded that routine debriefing within the first month of birth does not prevent psychological trauma in women following childbirth, it also surmised that due to the quality of studies included and a lack of homogeneity further high quality studies are needed to fully understand the role of postnatal debriefing.

There are, however, other therapeutic values inherent in utilising a debriefing style model post-partum, though we need to be careful that we are using the word *debriefing* correctly. Also, as practising clinicians will know, women do seek information regarding their birth events and want to discuss how they are feeling with an empathic listener. Yet there is little guidance as to how and when this should be done. We also know that women want more information, especially when complications occur (Dunning et al, 2016) and that they want to talk about their birth experience (Bailey & Price, 2008; Cooke & Stacey, 2003; Gamble, 2004; Inglis, 2002). In a meta-analysis Baxter et al (2014) found that women had a strong need to have their story heard, and valued being listened to by a midwife in a birth afterthoughts style session. Also whilst the consensus is that current models of debriefing do not prevent PTSD, Lavender and Walkinshaw's randomised control trial (1998) reported lower levels of depression and anxiety at three weeks post-partum when compared to a control group. In this study women were debriefed at two days following a normal birth. The intervention consisted of an interactive interview with a midwife discussing their labour, asking questions, and exploring their feelings. What we feel is important about this study is that, rather than being structured, the interviews were woman led rather than clinician led with hospital notes available throughout the interview. Furthermore, this type of active listening interaction which allows women to clarify their birth experience and 'make sense' of events with an empathic listener can be therapeutic in itself (Gamble, 2004), with the discussion providing validation, reassurance and support (Skibniewski-Woods, 2011). In a literature review exploring the perceptions of women accessing debriefing types of services post-partum, Baxter et al (2014) uses the term 'places a seal' over the birth experience, to describe the value of debriefing post-partum. From experience women often say 'I can move on now' after events have been clarified and better understood. Rather than placing a 'seal' over the experience which can be interpreted as shutting out the experience and risk maintaining symptoms of distress, we would suggest that the re-evaluation of events enables further processing and a chance to grow more from their experiences.

Two further studies have targeted intervention towards women who themselves *perceived* their birth experience as traumatic (Gamble et al, 2005; Meades et al, 2011) and this is important. In Chapter 2 we discussed that it is the woman's subjective experience of the birth that determines whether it activates the 'threat protection system' and is perceived as traumatic. Allocation in the Meades et al (2011) study was based on women self-referring to receive debriefing. Women ranged between twelve weeks and six years post-partum. Women reported significantly lower PTS symptoms at one month post-debrief. When women are able to self-select in this way there may already be a degree of psychological distress in relation to birth events. This is an important distinction and fits with the model of debriefing we would recommend. Used in this way, there is evidence that a debriefing service can be used as a stepped care model (Meades et al, 2011), with women being referred for additional psychology support as needed. This also fits with conclusions drawn from the first Cochrane review (Rose et al, 2002) that a more appropriate response to trauma events would be a 'screen and treat' model rather than a routine or universal offer. Sheen and Slade (2015) also conclude that targeted post-partum discussions for women who themselves perceive their birth as traumatic may hold some utility.

We feel self-selection is really important, in our experience clinicians often do not appreciate the validity of this approach, preferring instead to refer women who they perceive have had a traumatic birth. The problem with this approach is that it is clinician defined trauma when in fact trauma is 'in the eye of the beholder' and must be respected as such (Beck, 2004). Clinician-defined trauma also

- Ignores the experience of women who clinically appear to have had what professionals deem to be a typical or 'normal' experience but who nonetheless feel traumatised by birth.
- Fails to recognise the normal cognitive adaptive function of the human brain when dealing and recovering from unplanned events and trauma.
- Applies a label to the woman that she has had a 'traumatic birth' when in fact she may not be appraising her experience as traumatic.

We must remember that the majority of women will assimilate the experience of childbirth into their existing view of the world and maintain previous levels of emotional equilibrium. And as discussed in Chapter 2, women may actually experience personal growth, a greater appreciation of life and positive changes to functioning following a stressful and traumatic birth (Ayers, 2017; Joseph & Linley, 2006).

Listening to women in the post-partum period

In the first few days and weeks we would advocate using the word *defuse* adopted by Alexander (1998) to describe the practice of a midwife listening to a woman's birth narrative and then providing context and meaning. Many midwives routinely provide an opportunity to *defuse* the birth experience through routine postnatal care either in hospital or the community. Women want to talk about their birth experience, to synthesise events and importantly to have their experience validated (Baxter et al, 2014); it is also an important part of the transition to motherhood (Dahlen et al, 2010). Birth afterthoughts style sessions vary greatly across England, with many lacking consensus around referral criteria and training of staff, and are often under-resourced (Thomson & Garrett, 2019). Moving forwards, it is really important that we use the correct terminology, explaining events and circumstances surrounding the birth is one approach, but it is not a *debriefing* service unless a more structured model is used with the aim of facilitating cognitive adjustment, in addition many women who attend birth afterthoughts have not perceived their birth as traumatic or distressing but merely want to understand why for instance they had an emergency caesarean section. We recommend two different approaches depending on the time period. For the purposes of birth afterthoughts style sessions, which are delivered primarily by midwives, we would advocate the term suggested by Sheen and Slade (2015) of *childbirth review*, which as well as discussing elements of labour also addresses feelings and responses and avoids the inappropriate use of the term *debriefing*. We recommend that this takes place after six–eight weeks with no upward limit. Before six weeks we recommend that healthcare professionals act to *defuse* emotional distress and then refer on if distress has not diminished by six weeks.

Defusing events in the immediate post-partum period

As we have already discussed, in the first few days as the events of labour, birth and motherhood are being assimilated it is very common for women to be upset and tearful. A woman may also be experiencing flashbacks and nightmares surrounding her birth experience which she may articulate as being stressful and upsetting. In our experience midwives can feel ill-equipped to deal with these scenarios, often viewing them as evidence of psychological pathology, which they are not. This misappraisal may in part be a reflection on traditional pre-registration training and the limited amount of attention given to the role of the midwife within public health and specifically maternal mental health (McNeill et al, 2012). As explained above, the aim in these first few days and sometimes weeks, is to *defuse* not to diagnose psychological morbidity or to try and alleviate symptoms, referred to by Miller & Rollnick (2004) as the 'the righting reflex' (see Chapter 3). We would recommend three actions: listen, explain and normalise.

Listen: this is the most important action. Women need to feel able to express their feelings and emotions as they make sense of events. Try to avoid the need to 'fix' how she is feeling. It is ok for her not to feel ok this soon after birth; empathise, do not fix. Often on the postnatal wards, midwives will refer the woman to birth afterthoughts or request she has a *debrief* whilst still an in-patient to show they have acted to 'fix' what they perceive is a problem. However, as discussed in Chapter 1, the majority of women will assimilate and reconcile their experience over the first few weeks, with symptoms diminishing. Referring to a birth afterthoughts style session may be interpreted by the woman as evidence that her current emotional state is not normal

Explain: if there are gaps in memory or understanding provide simple explanations using jargon-free language. From experience women find holding onto information very difficult. Many women we see have had events explained to them in the first twenty-four to forty-eight hours of birth, yet very few retain the information in minds which are often fatigued and trying to process a multitude of various complex factors. As discussed in Chapter 1, how memory is encoded at this time will influence her cognitive synthesis of events and ultimately how she remembers her birth. It is really important therefore to avoid emotive language such as 'it's lucky you arrived when you did', which can be encoded by the mother as meaning 'I nearly lost my baby because I didn't seek help quickly enough'. We have experience of many women recounting this theme. Similarly, phrases such as 'we got him out in the nick of time' can be very upsetting to women as they try to make sense of events. A more useful phrase is 'we recognised that he needed some help and that is why we needed to …' It is useful if this is then backed up with 'it's not uncommon for babies to react like this in labour but they are very resilient and your baby is absolutely fine'. It is also important that the woman is allowed to frame her own birth experience. As discussed above labelling her birth for her as 'easy', 'quick' or 'traumatic' at this early stage is not helpful.

A frequent event that occurs immediately post-birth is post-partum haemorrhage (PPH). This event is usually accompanied by a frenzied rush of activity as staff rush into the room to enact first-line management and arrest the bleeding. This type of event is often recalled by women months after the birth, and even if the blood loss is between 500 mls and 1000 mls (this is not uncommon and not life threatening) and termed 'minor PPH' (RCOG, 2017) to that woman it can feel life threatening. Normalising this event, preferably whilst still in the birth room is really important: 'yes you lost more than is usual but this is not uncommon … we are all trained in what to do and we have lots of experience of it … it happens very quickly and that can feel frightening but you were always safe …'

It may be that intrapartum events have already been explained, but the ability to hold information can be limited so often women need further confirmation and reassurances. In pregnancy we expect women to have difficulty remembering events and in verbal recall, this is often referred to as 'baby brain' and is backed up by some neurobiological evidence (Glynn, 2010). In the post-partum period whilst overall cognitive performance improves, verbal recall memory remains poor (Glynn, 2010; Marrs et al, 2013).

Normalise: reassure her and her family that these feelings are normal at this point after childbirth, acknowledge her feelings/perception that the birth was stressful, frightening and/or traumatic, but do not collude in her interpretation. Provide reassurance that nightmares, flashbacks and frequent re-experiencing of events is common in the first few days and weeks. Explain to her that her brain is doing its job of trying to make sense of everything that has happened, and for most women by four–six weeks these feelings usually resolve. Remind her again that she and her baby are safe.

All of the above can be done by midwives on the wards and in community. Generally it requires a small amount of time and no additional specialist training, other than the ability to engage in active listening (see Chapter 3).

Providing a birth afterthoughts service

For women who want a more thorough discussion of events and to go through the notes we would advocate attending a birth afterthoughts session. We have drawn on Gamble and Creedy's (2009) post-partum counselling model and applied the principles of the Rogerian core conditions discussed in Chapter 3 to support exploration of feelings and responses and to support women in distress relating to their birth experience. Each woman will present with something different and it requires the skills of active listening, reflection on emotions, paraphrasing and conveying of genuine empathy, all of which form part of interpersonal counselling skills (Watkins, 2001). We have formulated our own communication model for use in a birth afterthoughts scenario to help guide the discussion, provide some structure for clinicians and to standardise the approach (see Box 4.1).

We would advocate that the model is used flexibly, depending on the type of service provision, clinician skill and needs of the woman. In our experience not all women want to vent feelings and emotions but want a factual account of what happened, often to fill in memory gaps and to understand implications for future pregnancies. The aim is to listen to the woman's story, her perception and her lived experience as this subjective experience will have formed her beliefs. Counselling theory uses the terms 'ventilation' and 'validation' of experience and this means simply allowing her to discuss her feelings and acknowledging them as real. In addition the model allows for memory gaps to be filled and to challenge negative emotions/self-beliefs formed through the woman's subjective experience. Working alongside a psychology service, we favour a stepped care model and advocate that the second part of the session should screen for symptoms of PTSD, and if positive refer for psychology assessment (see Chapter 5). Whilst we use the principles of person-centred counselling much of this can be learned without the need for a formal counselling qualification. We would advocate, however, that the service is delivered alongside psychological input with access to clinical supervision for the staff involved.

BOX 4.1 Five-Step Model for listening to women after childbirth

	Aim	*Content/actions*	*Example dialogue*
A Intro	Establishing a rapport and setting the scene	Introductions, length and purpose of session (see also Box 4.2 in Chapter 4)	'the purpose of this session is for you to talk through your labour and birth – is that what you were expecting today?' 'do you still feel ok to talk about this today?'
B Listen	Acknowledge the narrative and accept legitimacy of experience and feelings	Allow content of session to be set by the woman Encourage her to tell her story Open posture, be aware of body language Active listening, maintain eye contact Do not disagree or judge Clarify meaning if needed-try and keep interruptions to a minimal	'I have the medical notes here and we can use them later if there are parts you want to clarify, but first I am interested in your perspective, how it felt for you … where would you like to start?' 'When you say you were worried at the time what did you mean' 'yes we can clarify that later with the notes'
	Explore feelings and perceptions	Allow ventilation and exploration of lived experience Reflect understanding, use paraphrasing Validate emotional distress/perceived negative experience Identify 'hot spots'	'you said that the midwife kept leaving the room, how did that make you feel' 'I can see that you are very upset by that aspect' 'Is there one particular point in your experience that you keep going back to …?'
C Reflect & Reappraise	Clarify events, decisions and explain physiology of childbirth	Fill in memory gaps Gently address significant errors in narrative/assumed truth Explain rationale behind clinical decision making, and how the body works in labour Address any safety fears in labour – avoid language that further accentuates fears i.e. 'it's lucky you arrived when you did'	'I can understand that you feel you were left in labour for too long before the caesarean and you must have felt exhausted, let me explain what was happening …' 'I can see from the notes that you and your baby were never in danger, I understand you felt scared for your baby when the staff kept looking at the heart rate, baby's often show changes on the CTG and we don't always communicate to our best, but let me show you his other results that were all normal …'

	Challenge negative perceptions of self	Support women to feel positive about their bodies Reflect back on expressed feelings/ distress – normalise feeling of fear, lack of control	'there is nothing wrong with you or your body, childbirth can be unpredictable, you should be proud of what you achieved' 'don't forget you nurtured this baby for 9 months, you did everything you could to take care of your unborn baby, you already had a bond and a love for this baby, for some reason on this day he was in a hurry, but you still gave birth to him and you are still giving him everything he needs now to nurture him through his first few weeks and months, be proud of what you have done'
D Screen	Assess for birth trauma and postnatal depression	Avoidance-explore circumstances, what/ when Hyperarousal – explore behaviour Flashbacks – assess how often, when Check if having adequate sleep/rest Appetite-normal, supressed, over-eating	'you said that you were very emotional when you first arrived home and kept thinking about what happened, how are you feeling now …?' 'How did it feel coming back here today …' 'how are you finding being a new mother' or 'how is your relationship with [name of baby]
	Support networks	Social support available Involvement of health visitor, GP Permission to share with HV if appropriate	'are you getting out to baby clinics' 'have you joined any groups' 'is there anyone you feel you can talk to about your birth experience?' 'is there anyone you feel really understands how you feel about the birth?'
	Future pregnancies	Offer support for next time if available being sensitive to the context and readiness Explain options and choices for next birth	'you may not be thinking about this right now, but if you do think, later down the line about another pregnancy, we can offer …'
E Conclude	Closure and actions (if needed)	Re-affirm validity of the lived experience Apologise (if appropriate) for the emotional distress Take ownership of learning points/actions arising from the narrative	'We could have communicated with you better during your labour, I'm sorry that has been your experience and I am pleased that you feel you have a better understanding now' 'We always take feedback seriously; with your permission I would like to feed this back to …' Is there anything else that could have made your experience better?

Accessing a birth afterthoughts service

There is no agreed optimal timing for when women should access a birth afterthoughts session, with studies evidencing differing time limits depending on the sample population, methodology, intervention and measure (Sheen & Slade, 2015). In our own experience we recommend waiting until six–eight weeks post-partum. After that women should access the service whenever they feel ready (Bailey & Price, 2008; Inglis, 2002). The reason for recommending waiting until six–eight weeks is twofold: first, emotionally women are more able to synthesise information and the rawness of the birth experience has usually dulled making recall less stressful; second, symptoms such as flashbacks, nightmares and hyperarousal which can be expected within the first six weeks post-partum should have dissipated and if still present are indicative of possible PTSD; this then enables appropriate referral for psychology input. It also reduces the chance of disrupting normal psychological adaptation to events (Peeler et al, 2013).

Environment

The environment needs to facilitate discussion and disclosure and it is important that women feel at ease and unhurried. There also needs to be access to the medical notes which unless available electronically often precludes any environment outside of the hospital setting. One of the symptoms of PTSD can be that women will actively avoid triggers which remind them of childbirth (see Chapter 2). Some women will feel physically and emotionally unable to return to the hospital setting. In our experience, some will change their previous routines to actively avoiding walking or driving past the hospital. In such circumstances, home visiting or seeing in another venue may be necessary. Logistically depending on number of women accessing the service, ease of access to clinical notes and clinician time, a hospital-based service works well. In our experience for every 100 women referred, one woman will require a visit away from the hospital setting.

Pre-arrival

The most important aspect of this type of listening service is that the direction and content is directed by the woman and not by what we may think are the important aspects of her childbirth. To enable this we would advocate only a brief look at the clinical notes to ascertain the health of the baby, type of onset of labour, type of birth and length of stay and any neonatal input. If the notes are very unwieldy it may be useful to bookmark the stages of the journey for easy access later.

This approach is very normal for counsellors but can make clinicians feel vulnerable and risk looking inept; perhaps a reflection that clinicians prefer instead to be the knowledgeable practitioner, holding both the information and the control. We argue that in a person-centred approach the locus of control should be with the woman. When we read clinical notes, we make our own assumptions, we recognise scenarios and clinician names which then influences how we listen and respond to the woman's narrative. Also, the parts of the journey that are important to the woman may be very different to what we would interpret from the notes. One can spend half an hour scrutinising the management of the shoulder dystocia when in fact the woman has reconciled this part and wants to talk about her experience of induction of labour.

Post-partum childbirth review model (see Box 4.1)

A. Introduction

Establishing a rapport and setting the scene is important as women need to feel safe to talk through emotions and feelings. It is important that women also understand the aim of the session and to ensure it fits with what they are expecting. Counselling models include the term 'contract', which is used at the beginning to articulate the structure of the session. We would advocate a simple version which includes:

Purpose of session
Readiness to talk
Time available
Confidentiality

Whilst you may wish to adapt for different scenarios, having a script in mind which you use at the beginning of the session is useful for consistency, especially if there is a group of clinicians who deliver the same service. (An example is used in Box 4.2.) If a woman seems tentative or unsure where to start her narrative it is useful to ask an open question such as 'could you tell me about your pregnancy?' This is often a good way to start the conversation and is similar to the 'reverse funnel' as described in Chapter 3. It allows the woman to relax and for the discussion to move at a pace agreed by the woman towards the labour and birth narrative. This is usually the reason women have accessed birth afterthoughts and women can feel vulnerable and exposed, nervous of recalling their experience and their ability to maintain composure. Starting on more neutral ground can be useful. It is also useful to ask the woman what she wants to get out of the session, as this can provide a sense of how to structure the time available. For instance, she may they feel fine about how she was looked after on the labour ward but is upset at having been separated from her newborn immediately post-birth. We also recommend making your credentials and role clear to women. We would suggest that whilst practitioners may hold a counselling qualification this type of stand-alone session should not be interpreted as counselling. It utilises a person-centred approach but the facilitator is in the role of experienced clinical practitioner and not a counsellor.

BOX 4.2 Example of setting the scene

'The purpose of this session is for you to talk through your labour and birth, is that what you were expecting today? I have briefly looked at your clinical notes but I am more interested in your story – how it felt for you – do you still feel ok to talk about this today? We have one hour to talk everything through, I may make some notes as you talk but I don't keep these notes and at the end of the session we can discuss if you want your information to be shared, does that sound ok? Can you tell me what you would like to get out of this session …? Ok where would you like to start …?'

B. Listen

Acknowledge the narrative and accept legitimacy of experience and feelings. How women interpret their birth experience is uniquely insightful. Narratives offer a different lens and can be multi layered and rich in meaning (Borg Cunen et al, 2014). The woman's experience may not be how care was intended to be interpreted, and the care received may have followed all guidance. But what clinicians view as a successful birth will not always correspond to the woman's view of success (Lavender et al, 1999). In birth afterthoughts it must be interpreted and respected as the lived reality for that woman. In this way it becomes easier not to justify or defend clinical care and/or clinicians' behaviour, or to impose our interpretation of events onto the woman. This is not to say that falsehoods go unchallenged as these can be explored during the next stage of 'reflect and reappraise'.

As the woman tells her story, it is important to give her your full attention. Maintain open body language and eye contact. One of the hardest aspects of active listening can be to zone out all other thoughts and to just concentrate on the narrative and on her body language (see Chapter 3). Unless you need to clarify meaning, it is important to allow the woman to tell her story in full. Keep a note of any questions that arise or elements that you know need explaining. Use statements such as 'yes, I can answer that for you when we go through your notes', rather than disturbing the flow and taking over dialogue and control. It is not uncommon for women to feel tearful and upset as they talk through their experience. As empathic practitioners who experience women in emotional distress frequently in clinical practice, we are socialised to respond, to soothe and to give tactile reassurance. It is important, however, that this does not arrest or suppress the ventilation of emotions and feelings. It is important that these emotions are allowed to be vented. To enable this, one of the most useful skills a facilitator can have is to be comfortable with silence and able to tolerate a woman's distress without responding to the urge to close it down.

Explore feelings and perceptions. When the story is completed reflect understanding by paraphrasing certain elements that you have interpreted to be significant. This enables you to 'sense check' what you have heard. It also demonstrates to the woman that she has been heard and that you are engaged with her narrative (Fenwick et al, 2013; Gamble & Creedy, 2009). To give some understanding of appropriate responses see the example in Box 4.3, Jane attended a birth afterthoughts session four months after she gave birth to her first child. Her labour was induced for post-dates pregnancy, she had a normal vaginal birth but this was complicated by a post-partum haemorrhage. She struggled physically and emotionally in the weeks after the birth and had unreconciled emotions surrounding her induction experience.

BOX 4.3 Example of paraphrasing, ventilation and validation

Clinician: It sounds like you found the induction process very difficult and you felt alone as your husband was not there. You said that you felt unprepared for the induction and I could see you were upset when you talked about the midwife on night duty what was it that upset you about that part? [*paraphrasing and reflecting understanding*]

Jane: I didn't realise the pain would be so bad, I thought I could do it, but is was so painful, I was up and down all night, no one came to me, I hadn't slept, I was so tired, I asked the midwife if I could have something for the pain … she shrugged and said, well if you aren't coping you could have an injection … she made me feel like I was causing a fuss …

Clinician: it sounds like you felt she didn't recognise or respond to your distress? [*reflect meaning*]

Jane: No, I felt she dismissed me, I am a very strong person, I am not someone who complains, I know how busy the staff are but I went all night without asking for help,

I couldn't understand why it was so painful, I thought something must be wrong … [*ventilation of feelings*]

Clinician: what do you mean 'something was wrong'? [*reflecting meaning*]

Jane: I couldn't believe that this pain was normal … and so I was worried about what it was doing to my baby …

Clinician: I can understand why that must have been frightening, it sounds like you were seeking reassurance and support from the midwife, but you didn't feel you got any, and I am sorry that was your experience. [*validate emotional distress*]

C. Reflect and reappraise

Clarify events, decisions and explain physiology of childbirth. After the woman has told her story and you have explored *feelings and perceptions* from the 'touch points' in the journey, the parts that feel important to the woman will be evident. The medical notes have all the information to answer the clinical care aspects and as you articulate the woman's actual journey you can explain the uncertainties and misinformation that the woman has expressed in her narrative. Alongside this, it is useful to weave in what was happening in the body and explain the physiology of labour.

In Jane's case (Box 4.3), it was important for her to understand from a clinician perspective that induction of labour (IOL) is very different from spontaneous labour and to assure her that the pain intensity she felt is not because she was weak but because IOL is an artificial process that is usually interpreted by women as excessively painful. As clinicians we see the IOL process daily but women have no reference point and no comparison. Jane also expressed that she was concerned her baby was at risk during the process, it was important for her to understand that well-grown term babies are resilient to the stress of labour and to reassure her using clinical markers from the medical notes that her baby was never in danger. As part of the dialogue we also talked about how hard it can be to be in labour on the antenatal ward during the night without the support of a partner and how this impacted on her ability to cope. We also talked through changes that now support partners to stay on the wards as other women too have found this isolation unsettling and we have listened.

We also feel honesty is very important. One of the recurring narratives that women talk to us about pertain to the latent phase of labour. This is not surprising, it is a contentious, under-researched area (Janssen et al, 2009), linked to an increase in intervention (Cheng et al, 2010; Lundgren et al, 2013; McNiven et al, 1998), and is viewed negatively by women (Carlsson et al, 2009). In our experience when you explain the difficulties with the latent phase, such as the lack of research and the complexity of the decision making that can be involved, then women are generally more accepting. Labour and birth are not a simplistic mechanistic system that starts at A and travels seamlessly to B. We are still debating at what point latent phase becomes active phase (Hundley et al, 2017) and in our experience women find this detail useful in assimilating their experience. To reflect on this, we can only assume that there is value in understanding that labour and birth are not an exact science and that perhaps this adjusts their perceived view that we did not care or that what happened was due to an error in care.

During this part of the discussion it important to fill in any gaps and to clarify actual timings of events which often have been encoded inaccurately due to high stress levels at the time. For women who required a general anaesthetic and caesarean section, there may be no memory and often the first memory is of waking up to find a baby in a cot. Women are often keen to know what was happening. In other areas of medicine, for instance intensive care, diaries are kept and staff or relatives record events whilst the patient is unconscious, and this has found to be valuable when used as part of a later discussion once the patient has regained consciousness (O'Gara & Pattison, 2016). One of the methods we find useful is to produce a time line of events for women, including exactly what was happening to their baby during the birth in theatre, who was holding him, caring for him, and describing if he was crying or quiet. In addition, it is helpful to use any photos that were taken in the first few hours and assimilate these with the time line. Women often have no recollection of their early post-partum recovery; with the general anaesthetic still wearing off they often have no memory of events such as early skin-to-skin contact whilst still in the recovery room. Using a timeline helps to show that actually skin to skin happened less than an hour after birth. Of course, events are not always so straightforward and women can often experience extreme emotions stemming from the fact that they 'missed out' on their baby being born. This can relate to the sense of grief described in Chapter 1. For some women there is a sense of detachment that can have far reaching effects (see Helen's experience in Case Study 4.1). Helen was seen in birth afterthoughts at twelve weeks post-partum; she screened positive for PTSD and after psychology input was able to enjoy a very healthy and happy relationship with her babies.

CASE STUDY 4.1 Helen's experience

Helen had a long and difficult journey which started with being unable to conceive naturally and then after repeated treatments found she was pregnant with twins. After the initial shock she was starting to enjoy her pregnancy. Then at thirty-two weeks the pregnancy was suddenly over and she started to labour. Due to complications she was rushed to theatre and felt divorced from proceedings. Helen recalled 'I felt I was no longer present in the room and my body was being used for some experiment' with a screen in place she was unable to see her twins being born and she could not recall any dialogue to tell her that the twins were OK. Later she was wheeled around to the neonatal unit and she said 'they could have been anybody's'. This was compounded by Helen's feeling of powerlessness as a mother as the babies continued to be cared for on the neonatal unit 'I felt like a visitor … they belong to special care, you can't pick them up, change their nappy – they are not yours'.

Challenge negative perceptions of self. Through working emotionally with women after childbirth, you start to see the consequences of self-doubt, guilt and often the manifestation of shame which we have discussed in Chapter 2. In this part of the session we have a valuable window in which to offer her an alternative lens. In our experience women are often unaware of how clinical aspects such as a baby in the occipital-posterior position (baby lying back to back in-utero) or interventions such as IOL and artificially breaking the forewater's can have on labour progress, pain and the choices that are made at the time. We often use a doll and pelvis to explain what has happened and to articulate just how hard labour can be under these circumstances. It is evident in birth afterthoughts sessions that women often judge themselves harshly based on distorted thinking and a lack of understanding (Murphy et al, 2003) and can be left with feelings of self-blame (Elmir et al, 2010) for a subjectively imposed interpretation that is often unrelated to actual events (Storksen et al, 2013). Gently addressing these negative beliefs and feelings of self-blame is important in supporting a more positive reappraisal of the birth and role therein of the woman (Gamble & Creedy, 2009).

One of the most common questions we hear is 'could I have done anything differently?' It is important that women understand that even if we could change one component of their journey, that is, arriving at hospital earlier a different outcome is not certain and may have altered another component in the journey/narrative. It is also useful to affirm that their decision making at the time was good given the information or presenting facts at the time, affirmations are important and form part of the OARS model of communication, discussed in Chapter 3. Sometimes you can sense that a woman may be struggling to verbalise feelings of guilt and depending on the scenario it can be useful to articulate 'you do know that none of this is your fault' and see how she responds. It is also useful to articulate all the positive and amazing things she has done to ensure the security of her newborn through pregnancy, labour and post-partum. This might be nurturing her baby through a healthy pregnancy, enjoying skin-to-skin contact and all the benefits this brings, establishing breastfeeding or just providing a loving and secure attachment. We find this approach particularly important when after an emergency caesarean section, women verbalise that they feel 'robbed' of a vaginal birth. This is usually accompanied by a sense of guilt as they have a healthy child which they feel gives them no right to grieve for the unmet expectation of vaginal birth. The fact that she has been able to articulate this is very important and the most important act is to listen and to empathise. There are no easy glib answers to make this adjustment easier. It is useful however to tell her that many women feel the same mix of disappointment mixed with guilt. How you answer will depend of course on the scenario and needs to be tailored to the woman's experience. From a psychological perspective it is about how much value someone attaches to this one particular experience or emotion. Feelings and emotions don't always make sense; women often say 'I know deep down it doesn't matter but I can't help how it makes me feel …' Women find it useful to understand that there isn't really a rational answer and that it is OK to just feel the grief, to allow it and to work through it, as many women do. Stott (2007) refers to this as the 'heart-head lag' a dissociation between rational beliefs and how it feels. Box 4.4 gives an example of how we might typically respond, elements of which can be adapted and tailored.

BOX 4.4 Example of challenging negative perceptions

Clinician: I hear this so many times from women, I promise you are not alone. What always astounds me is how women forget just how strong, brave and amazing they are … you have nurtured this baby through early pregnancy to full term, you have loved him unconditionally, paid attention to his movements, learnt all you can to ensure you can be prepared and well equipped for his every need. You coped amazingly in labour, your first experience of labour, you gave him skin to skin and kept him warm, you have managed to come through the early days of exhaustion, pain and emotional upheaval to be able to give your baby the most important start to his life, that of love and security and additionally you are still breastfeeding. All of that is amazing. So it depends just how much importance you choose to attach to the one element of that total experience, the fact that your baby birthed through his mother's abdomen rather than her vagina or you could choose to attach importance to the rest of journey and what you are continuing to provide now.

Providing women with positive feedback about their role in the journey of their baby from conception to birth and post-partum is an important part of enabling women to re-align their feelings and re-assimilate their labour and birth experience. Unresolved negative appraisals of birth can affect a woman's emotional wellbeing in the post-partum period and also her sense of self (Waldenstrom et al, 2004). It can also affect how she sees herself as a mother (Larkin et al, 2009).

Box 4.3 discusses Jane's IOL experience, Jane was happy with her care on the labour ward including the management of her post-partum haemorrhage. She described feeling 'safe' and that 'everyone knew what they doing'. The next part of Jane's narrative was her postnatal journey which she found much harder than she imagined and blamed herself with feelings of inadequacy. Having clarified events around her labour and birth it was clear from a clinician perspective that Jane's description of her post-partum journey was entirely normal especially given the fact her haemoglobin (Hb) on discharge was just 88 g/dL (post-partum anaemia is defined as an Hb <100 g/dL affects and symptoms include fatigue, breathlessness and dizziness; RCOG, 2015). Through discussion it emerged that Jane was judging herself against her sister who also had a normal birth and was 'up and dressed' and receiving visitors on the second day. This was her only reference point for post-partum recovery and it challenged her self-identify as a resilient and strong woman. Her own experience was one of physical exhaustion and emotional fragility that lasted for weeks. We talked through the physical aspects of her induction of labour, birth, post-partum haemorrhage and subsequent low Hb. In addition we talked through the emotional impact of first-time motherhood and breastfeeding with a low Hb. Jane had no understanding that her low Hb was responsible for her feelings of inertia and difficulties establishing breastfeeding, this lack of knowledge is reflected in research around women's experience of post-partum haemorrhage (Dunning et al, 2016). We talked through who decides what is normal post-birth and that as clinicians, given her childbirth experience, her post-partum behaviour is seen as entirely normal. We also talked through her perceived sense of failure and offered an alternative view: she had laboured under difficult circumstances with little or no sleep; her body had responded really well to the induction process and she laboured brilliantly; despite her fatigue she pushed her baby out with no assistance; despite her low Hb she had succeeded at breastfeeding and she was providing everything her newborn needed (love, security, food, comfort). Understanding that as clinicians her postnatal journey was very normal was important for Jane. This new information enabled her to reappraise her own subjective birth appraisal, modify her feelings/beliefs and actually feel a sense of achievement.

D. Screen

Assess for birth trauma and postnatal depression. In Chapter 2 we discussed the symptom recognition for PTSD. As clinicians and not psychologists we recommend a fluid, person-centred approach to the assessing of symptoms rather than utilising a formal trauma checklist. The aim is to assess if symptoms are evident and to then refer for further psychology assessment.

During the narrative phase high levels of emotional distress and anxiety on recalling events are often apparent. These have been coined 'hotspots' and refer to memories which cause the highest levels of emotional distress (Holmes et al, 2005) As discussed earlier obstetric interventions, or our own interpretation of what appears to be a traumatic birth are unreliable as a marker for PTSD. This is because 'hotspots' are strongly linked to interpersonal difficulties during birth, commonly feeling ignored, unsupported or abandoned and these are the strongest predictors of PTSD (Harris & Ayers, 2012) (see Rebecca's experience in Case Study 4.2).

CASE STUDY 4.2 Rebecca's experience

Rebecca had unresolved feelings fourteen months after her first birth. She recalled that labour started well and when she came to hospital, she was pleased that she was already 5 cm dilated. After some time her labour slowed and then stalled, she had further intervention to speed up labour but she started to feel that she was failing and that she couldn't continue. She felt alone and there was a lack of appropriate information for Rebecca to be able to make sense of how her labour was progressing, leaving her feeling vulnerable and scared. Her hotspot recollection was very vivid, she was laid on the bed, she remembers the exact time of 0610 and thinking 'if there was a button to take my life, I would press it now'. This repeating image was hugely distressing for Rebecca and one she knew she needed to address before she could try to conceive again.

How women react at the time of these events occurring or just after is important. Some women describe peritraumatic dissociation which enables a woman to detach herself from the trauma (Seng et al, 2009). See Chapter 2 for further discussion and a case study illustrating this. Though not a common occurrence during a birth afterthoughts session, this type of 'out of body' experience is considered an important of predictor of PTSD (Harris & Ayers, 2012).

In our stepped care model we recommend assessing for the following PTS symptoms: *re-experiencing the trauma*, *avoidance of trigger stimuli* and *hyperarousal.* The presence of all three is strongly suggestive of PTSD (see Chapter 2). This can be woven into the narrative rather than asking closed, specific questions. It is important to verify if symptoms have worsened or diminished following birth and the frequency of symptoms. Our model is based on seeing women after at least six weeks so that a clinician can appropriately *assess* for PTS symptoms and then refer to a psychology team for a comprehensive formulation of how the woman's presentation is consistent with a diagnosis of PTSD and the associated factors.

Re-experiencing the trauma

This usually takes the form of the following:

- Recurrent intrusive thoughts/recollections
- Flashbacks-being back in the event
- Recurrent nightmares
- Physiological reactivity

Intrusive thoughts are uncontrollable unconscious ruminative reflections that frequently push themselves into conscious thought, whereas flashbacks feel like being back in the event including feeling the same sensations and emotions. Listening to women as they describe emotionally charged accounts of their perceived care and birth experience can be unsettling. Often the memories are very raw and graphic in nature and women can sometimes describe sensory flashbacks as part of their re-experiencing (see Heather's experience in Case Study

4.3). Heather attended birth afterthoughts after the birth of her first child she had been on the midwife-led unit, her labour was complicated by a prolonged first stage of labour and when she left the pool she struggled to cope. She was able to vividly recall her journey from the midwife-led unit to the obstetric theatre for an emergency caesarean under spinal anaesthesia.

CASE STUDY 4.3 Heather's experience

'… I remember hearing someone screaming and then I realised it was me … my mum had been waiting outside the room whilst they examined me … I will never forget the look on her face as they wheeled me half naked down the corridor to the theatre … I did that to her … I must have still been screaming when we arrived in the theatre as I heard someone say "looks like we have a screamer" … I was so frightened … so scared … why did he say that … at night when its quiet and I am laid on my back, I am back in that theatre, I can hear the sounds and I lose the feeling in my legs again, it's like I can't move and I can feel a soreness in my hand where the drip is …'

Heather was experiencing these sensory flashbacks during the night when the house was quiet and she couldn't pre-occupy herself with physically demanding tasks. In our experience this is a common pattern for re-experiencing the trauma. Commonly with PTS symptoms women will describe situations, sounds, sights, smells and places that trigger the painful memory. These triggers are an important factor in the assessment of PTSD. Commonly expressed *triggers* are as follows: seeing other pregnant women; seeing or hearing birth stories in the media; revisiting hospitals; attending clinic appointments; and going to the GP. Sometimes the trigger relates directly to a sensory aspect of the experience, such as the sound of a 999 siren after an emergency transfer from a homebirth, or it can be related to a specific time of day that is associated with a traumatic memory.

As the trigger brings back the memories some women can experience a physical reaction known as physiological reactivity. This can take many forms but commonly sweating, palpitations, hyperventilating, feeling frozen to the spot and panic attacks.

Ask
'How often do you think back to the birth now?'
'When do these memories occur?'
'Is there a certain point in your labour that you keep remembering?'
'Is there anything that triggers your memories?'

Avoidance of trauma-related stimuli

In order to protect themselves from remembering the trauma, women will describe actively avoiding certain situations, places or people which act as trigger. It is not uncommon for women to avoid busy shopping centres where they are likely to see other pregnant women or to decline social situations, including integrating into 'baby groups' and other sources of social support for new mothers. Avoidant behaviour can also prevent women from discussing their birth experience with friends or discussing the psychological impact with professionals and can leave some women potentially isolated (Byrne et al, 2017). It can also impact on relationships, with women avoiding intimacy and sexual intercourse due to fear of another pregnancy or triggering memories (Elmir et al, 2010). In the longer term, there can be an avoidance of future pregnancy (Borg Cunen et al, 2014).

Ask
'How did you feel coming back here (hospital) today?'
'Are there any situations that are making you feel particularly anxious?'
'How often are you leaving the house/how does it make you feel?'

Hyperarousal

Symptoms of hyperarousal include:

Difficulty with falling or staying sleeping
Feeling irritable or angry
Trouble concentrating
Being overly alert or jumpy

Hyperarousal symptoms post-partum are often the most common feature within a women's narrative, and is known to be more common post-partum than the experiences of *re-experiencing* and *avoidance* (Ayers et al, 2009). Women are often fatigued and sleep deprived and are on high alert to the needs of their baby, hard wired to respond. In one study, hyperarousal symptoms were experienced by 50 per cent of women who had non-traumatic birth (Ayers et al, 2015).

Discussing these can be important for assessing other relational aspects with her family and available social support.

Ask
'How well are you sleeping?'
'How are things with your partner?'
'How does it feel being a mum for the first time?'
'How is your relationship now with [baby name]?'
'Do you have anyone you feel safe opening up to about how you are feeling?'

Providing a safe space for the woman answer honestly about how she feels as a mum or her relationship with her baby is important. Whilst the evidence linking PTSD with delayed or absent mother–infant attachment is limited (McKenzie-Mcharg et al, 2015), this is often due to the presence of comorbid depressive symptomology in many women experiencing PTSD, making it difficult to know which is the main contributory factor (Williams et al, 2016).

Postnatal depression

Postnatal depression is known to affect areas of parenting including a reduced responsiveness to infant cues (Murray et al, 2010) and negative child outcomes across cognitive, behavioural and emotional purviews (Stein et al, 2014).

Postnatal depression is still under-detected and under-reported (Johnson et al, 2015). The birth afterthoughts session gives women the opportunity to express feelings, emotions and insecurities to an attentive and empathic healthcare professional. These elements are considered important by women when disclosing information about mental health (Poole et al, 2006). See also Chapter 3 for a discussion on suicide risk assessment.

Support networks. Social support available in the perinatal period plays a significant role in improving maternal mental health and in the normal adaptation to motherhood (Li et al, 2017). It is important that women do experience these social interactions as supportive, and not as additional stress (for example, spending time with family who do not understand or tolerate how she is feeling will not be experienced as supportive for a woman who is struggling). It is the quality of support, rather than its presence or absence that determines its usefulness. During this part of the session we recommend a short enquiry around the following, and referring back to the health visiting team and/or GP if any concerns:

Availability of partner and family support
Peer groups and friends
Attendance at mother and baby groups
Engagement with health visitor team and GP
Ask
'How are you finding getting out and about with a little one?'
'What opportunities and places do you have where you live?'
'How is your partner feeling?'

Future pregnancies. The level of discussion around future pregnancies will need to be tailored to each individual woman with sensitivity around current level of distress and the nature of events during labour. There is evidence that women who have a negative birth experience may avoid future pregnancies or delay childbearing (Borg Cunen et al, 2014) and the evidence is inconclusive as to whether debriefing postnatally will reduce the fear of childbirth in the longer term (Kershaw et al, 2005). It can be used to further reinforce to the women that she has not failed or that there is nothing wrong with her body. It also allows women to ask questions about how she should approach her next birth and to be able to feel a sense of control about the future (Gamble & Creedy, 2009). It is also useful to mention that often emotions and anxieties can become heightened again during pregnancy and that this is entirely normal. For that reason, we offer another opportunity to talk in a subsequent pregnancy (see Chapter 7). Women should be reassured that their labour management in the next pregnancy can be flexible with shared decision making to address previous negative experiences and anxieties.

E. Conclude

Closure and actions. This is a chance to re-affirm the validity of her lived experience and if necessary, apologise for any emotional distress that has been caused as a result of *perceived* negative staff responses. This is not to say that you are criticising your colleagues, you are merely validating what she has perceived. We would suggest saying 'I am sorry that you felt her response was unkind.' If there was a delay in a period care it is acceptable to say 'I am sorry that this was your experience' or agree that, with better communication, events may have been easier to understand at the time: 'I am sorry, we could have communicated with you better during your labour.' Women usually react very positively to this kind of empathic understanding and to an apology. Take ownership of learning points/actions there will be some repeated narratives from women that lend themselves to service change (see Chapter 8). In other cases, there may be individual learning for clinicians to understand how the woman has interpreted events. Women are often keen that feedback, good and bad, is actually actioned following the meeting. If referral for further psychology assessment is warranted and accepted by the woman, the process should be discussed and confirmed before she leaves.

Understanding the father's experience

Whilst a birth afterthoughts session is aimed towards the woman's narrative and experience of birth, birth partners too will also accompany mothers to a session, often though not exclusively this is the father of the baby.

We acknowledge that this reflects a heteronormative culture and are not intending to support heterosexual family discourses as the only 'reality' and 'truth' of our social system (Foucault, 2002). As healthcare professionals it is important that we do not assume sexual orientation and support with acceptance and without judgement (McManus et al, 2006). There is a growing evidence base evaluating lesbian mothers' experience of maternity care with studies showing encouragingly that the experience is positive (Cherguit et al, 2013; Larsson & Dykes, 2009). There is also still a lack of research exploring other diverse groups within both the birth trauma literature (McKenzie-Mcharg et al, 2015) in particular, lesbian experiences of childbirth and parenting (McManus et al, 2006), and on co-mother experiences (Cherguit et al, 2013) and other LGBTQ+ experiences within maternity. It is interesting to note that in Cherguit et al's (2013) study lesbian co-mothers felt they were afforded more privileges than most fathers because they were female, able to share experiences, build allegiances through the shared identity as a woman within a women-centred maternity service. In contrast, Steen et al's (2011) study of fathers' encounters with maternity care described them as feeling marginalised and occupying an undefined space as 'not-patient' and 'not-visitor'.

In the UK, access to perinatal mental health services for fathers and the importance of strengthening the mental health for both parents are being addressed in national policy (NHS England, 2019) through the development of outreach clinics, with further aims to expand access to psychological therapies for parent–infant, couple, co-parenting and family interventions. When fathers attend birth afterthoughts it is useful to understand how they experience labour, the emotions and difficulties they may still be experiencing and how this can impact on the parent–infant relationship and the emotional wellbeing of the mother.

An interesting analysis by Chapman (1992) of the role identification and engagement of men during the labour process describes fathers as acting within three domains (see Box 4.5). This active versus inactive role of fathers during birth has been repeated in more recent evidence and has been shown to relate to their evaluation of the birth process (Longworth et al, 2015).

BOX 4.5 Role identification of fathers in labour (Chapman, 1992)

Role	*Behaviours*
Coach	Active role, high degree of engagement, see themselves as leaders within the experience and are highly supportive of their partners
Teammate	Active role, see themselves as a helper responding to requests made by their partner
Witness	Inactive role, see themselves as an observer, often looking for a distraction i.e. watching television or reading

Fathers have a strong desire to be present at the birth of their child (Johansson et al, 2015) but need *information* and *support* from midwives during the labour event (Longworth & Kingdon, 2011). When this occurs, they feel safe and able to play a more active role in the labour room (Johansson et al, 2015) and they are also highly likely to describe the birth experience as positive (Alio et al, 2011; Hildingsson et al, 2011). When these two components are missing, it can lead to stress and anxiety (Elmir & Schmied, 2016; Johansson et al, 2015) as well as feelings of anger, fear and helplessness (Vallin et al, 2019), which may be expressed during the birth afterthoughts session.

When a labour becomes complicated and obstetric intervention is required, communication becomes even more important. In these circumstances, fathers may try to make sense of events by attempting to read the faces and gestures of professionals in attendance (Premberg et al, 2011). Often, however, partners feel abandoned and fearful for the health of their partner and baby (Lindberg & Engström, 2013). In an attempt to maintain the focus of attention on the woman and not themselves, men will often try to conceal their own feelings and remain calm (Etheridge & Slade, 2017). When separation from their partner is required, the feelings of exclusion, fear and abandonment can be heightened (Vallin et al, 2019).

We have listened to men during birth afterthoughts sessions recall vivid scenes of being left in the room 'holding the baby' with blood evident on the floor, and this type of scenario has been repeated in studies exploring the experiences of fathers (Dunning et al, 2016). Often in the immediacy of events, with the best intentions staff have to prioritise the woman. But repeated stories like these that can be used to change practice locally (see Chapter 8). Understanding how men may have felt during labour may be useful in explaining their demeanour and behaviour during a birth afterthoughts session. Certainly when partners attend they usually want information; some express unresolved anger and disappointment; and some can appear withdrawn. A dominant theme in the narratives we hear is that men feel they have let their partners down or somehow colluded in interventions by not speaking up (Longworth et al, 2015). Psychological distress in men including birth trauma is becoming increasingly recognised (Hinton et al, 2014). This is important as it may affect the amount of emotional support they are able to provide to their partner postpartum, which can in turn affect levels of PTS and depression in women (Iles et al, 2011). Psychological distress in partners can be evident in a birth afterthoughts session and whilst we can signpost to services, the difficulty is that men are less likely to seek help and support (Jessop & Fox, 2011).

Interventions in the future need to ensure more support for the psychological health of men, especially when birth has not been straightforward. When a father feels able to provide emotional as well as physical support it promotes a more positive child birth experience for both parents and can improve and bolster a sense of shared responsibility towards the infant (Alio et al, 2011; Awad & Bühling, 2011). This demonstrates the value of clinicians engaging with fathers during pregnancy to prepare them for the process of childbirth and arguably to give them access to information via birth afterthoughts.

Conclusion

Women present with a myriad of difference experiences and it is difficult to explore all scenarios. The above is intended to be used as a guide, the sessions need to be reflexive and iterative and we would recommend not sticking rigidly to a script or a tick box style assessment. Having an evidence-based framework enables healthcare practitioners to feel confident in implementing or redesigning listening services for women post-partum, services women want and value. In addition, listening to women after childbirth offers clinicians a chance to view practice from an alternative lens, to deepen understanding and to reflect on our practice.

References

Alexander, J. (1998). Confusingly debriefing and defusing postnatally: The need for clarity of terms, purpose and value. *Midwifery*, 14, 122–124.

Alio, A., Mbah, A., Grunsten, R. & Salihu, H. (2011). Teenage pregnancy and the influence of paternal involvement on fetal outcomes. *J Pediatr Adolesc Gynecol*, 24(6), 404–409.

Audit Commission (1997). *First class delivery: Improving maternity services in England and Wales.* London: Audit Commission.

Awad, O. & Bühling, K. (2011). Fathers in the delivery room: Results of a survey. *Geburtshilfe Frauenheilkd*, 71, 511–517.

Ayers, S. (2017). Birth trauma and post-traumatic stress disorder: The importance of risk and resilience. *Journal of Reproductive and Infant Psychology*, 35(5), 427–430.

Ayers, S., Claypool, J. & Eagle, A. (2006). What happens after a difficult birth? Postnatal debriefing services. *British Journal of Midwifery*, 14(3), 157–161.

Ayers, S., Harris, R., Sawyer, A., Parfitt, Y. & Ford, E. (2009). Posttraumatic stress disorder after childbirth: Analysis of symptom presentation and sampling. *Journal of Affective Disorders*, 119(1–3), 200–204.

Ayers, S., Wright, D. B. & Ford, E. (2015). Hyperarousal symptoms after traumatic and nontraumatic births. *Journal of Reproductive and Infant Psychology*, 33(3), 282–293.

Bailey, M. & Price (2008). Exploring womens experiences of a Birth Afterthoughts service. *Evidence-based Midwifery*, 6, 52–58.

Bastos, M. H., Furuta, M., Small, R., McKenzie-McHarg, K. & Bick, D. (2015). Debriefing interventions for the prevention of psychological trauma in women following childbirth. *Cochrane Database of Systematic Reviews* (4).

Baxter, J. D., McCourt, C. & Jarrett, P. M. (2014). What is current practice in offering debriefing services to post partum women and what are the perceptions of women in accessing these services: A critical review of the literature. *Midwifery*, 30(2), 194–219.

Beck, T. C. (2004). Birth trauma: In the eye of the beholder. *Nursing Research,* 53(1), 28–35. doi:10.1097/00006199-200401000-00005.

Borg Cunen, N., McNeill, J. & Murray, K. (2014). A systematic review of midwife-led interventions to address post partum post-traumatic stress. *Midwifery*, 30(2), 170–184.

Brewin, C. R., Scragg, P., Robertson, M., Thompson, M., D'Ardenne, P. & Ehlers, A. (2008). Promoting mental health following the London bombings: A screen and treat approach. *Journal of Traumatic Stress*, 21(1), 3–8.

Byrne, V., Egan, J., Mac Neela, P. & Sarma, K. (2017). What about me? The loss of self through the experience of traumatic childbirth. *Midwifery*, 51, 1–11.

Carlsson, I. M., Hallberg, L. R. & Odberg Pettersson, K. (2009). Swedish women's experiences of seeking care and being admitted during the latent phase of labour: a grounded theory study. *Midwifery*, 25(2), 172–180.

Chapman, L. (1992). Expectant fathers' roles during labor and birth. *J Obstet Gynecol Neonatal Nurs*, 21(2), 114–120.

Cheng, Y. W., Shaffer, B. L., Bryant, A. S. & Caughey, A. B. (2010). Length of the first stage of labor and associated perinatal outcomes in nulliparous women. *Obstetrics & Gynecology*, 116(5), 1127–1135.

Cherguit, J., Burns, J., Pettle, S. & Tasker, F. (2013). Lesbian co-mothers' experiences of maternity healthcare services. *J Adv Nurs*, 69(6), 1269–1278.

Cooke, M. & Stacey, T. (2003). Differences in the evaluation of postnatal midwifery support by multiparous and primiparous women in the first two weeks after birth. *Australian Midwifery*, 16(3), 18–24.
Dahlen, H. G., Barclay, L. M. & Homer, C. S. (2010). Processing the first birth: Journeying into 'motherland'. *J Clin Nurs*, 19(13–14), 1977–1985.
Dunning, T., Harris, J. & Sandall, J. (2016). Women and their birth partners' experiences following a primary postpartum haemorrhage: A qualitative study. *BMC Pregnancy and Childbirth*, 16(80).
Dyregov, A. (1989). Caring for helpers in disaster situations: Psychological debriefing. *Disaster Management*, 2(1), 25–30.
Elmir, R. & Schmied, V. (2016). A meta-ethnographic synthesis of fathers' experiences of complicated births that are potentially traumatic. *Midwifery*, 32, 66–74.
Elmir, R., Schmied, V., Wilkes, L. & Jackson, D. (2010). Women's perceptions and experiences of a traumatic birth: A meta-ethnography. *Journal of Advanced Nursing*, 66(10), 2142–2153.
Etheridge, J. & Slade, P. (2017). "Nothing's actually happened to me": The experiences of fathers who found childbirth traumatic. *BMC Pregnancy and Childbirth*, 17(1), 80.
Fenwick, J., Gamble, J., Creedy, D., Barclay, L., Buist, A. & Ryding, E. L. (2013). Women's perceptions of emotional support following childbirth: a qualitative investigation. *Midwifery*, 29(3), 217–224.
Foucault, M. (2002). *The birth of the clinic* (1st edn). London: Routledge.
Fullerton, C., Ursano, R., Vance, K. & Wang, L. (2000). Debriefing following trauma. *Psychiatric Quarterly*, 71(3), 259–276.
Gamble, J., Creedy, D., Moyle, W., Webster, J., McAllister, M. & Dickson, P. (2005). Effectiveness of a counseling intervention after a traumatic childbirth: A randomized controlled trial. *Birth – Issues in Perinatal Care*, 32(1), 11–19.
Gamble, J. & Creedy, D. K. (2009). A counselling model for postpartum women after distressing birth experiences. *Midwifery*, 25(2), e21–30.
Gamble, J. C. D. (2004). Content and processes of postpartum counseling after a distressing birth experience: A review. *Birth*, 31(3), 213–218.
Glynn, L. M. (2010). Giving birth to a new brain: Hormone exposures of pregnancy influence human memory. *Psychoneuroendocrinology*, 35(8), 1148–1155.
Greenberg, N., Langston, V., Everitt, B., Iversen, A. C., Fear, N. T., Jones, N. & Wessely, S. C. (2010). A cluster randomized controlled trial to determine the efficacy of Trauma Risk Management (TRiM) in a military population. *Journal of Traumatic Stress*, 23(4), 430–436.
Harris, R. & Ayers, S. (2012). What makes labour and birth traumatic? A survey of intrapartum 'hotspots'. *Psychology and Health*, 27(10), 1166–1177.
Hildingsson, I., Cederlof, L. & Widen, S. (2011). Fathers' birth experience in relation to midwifery care. *Women Birth*, 24(3), 129–136.
Hinton, L., Locock, L. & Knight, M. (2014). Partner experiences of "near-miss" events in pregnancy and childbirth in the UK: A qualitative study. *PLoS One*, 9(4), e91735.
Holmes, E. A., Grey, N. & Young, K. A. D. (2005). Intrusive images and "hotspots" of trauma memories in posttraumatic stress disorder: An exploratory investigation of emotions and cognitive themes. *Journal of Behavior Therapy and Experimental Psychiatry*, 36(1), 3–17.
Hundley, V., Way, S., Cheyne, H., Janssen, P., Gross, M. & Spiby, H. (2017). Defining the latent phase of labour: is it important? *Evidence Based Midwifery*, 15(3), 89–94.
Iles, J., Slade, P. & Spiby, H. (2011). Posttraumatic stress symptoms and postpartum depression in couples after childbirth: The role of partner support and attachment. *J Anxiety Disord*, 25(4), 520–530.
Inglis, S. (2002). Accessing a debriefing service following birth. *British Journal of Midwifery*, 10(6), 368–371.
Janssen, P., Nolan, M. L., Spiby, H., Green, J., Gross, M. M., Cheyne, H., Hundley, V., Rijnders, M., De Jonge, A. & Buitendijk, S. (2009). Roundtable Discussion: Early Labor: What's the Problem? *Birth*, 36(4), 332–339.
Jessop, E. & Fox, P. (2011). 'What about then men?' Supporting fathers through birth trauma. *J Reproductive Infant Psychol*, 29(3), 25–26.

Johansson, M., Fenwick, J. & Premberg, A. (2015). A meta-synthesis of fathers' experiences of their partner's labour and the birth of their baby. *Midwifery*, 31(1), 9–18.

Johnson, A. R., Edwin, S., Joachim, N., Mathew, G., Ajay, S. & Joseph, B. (2015). Postnatal depression among women availing maternal health services in a rural hospital in South India. *Pakistan Journal of Medical Sciences*, 31(2), 408–413.

Joseph, S. & Linley, P. A. (2006). Growth following adversity: Theoretical perspectives and implications for clinical practice. *Clinical Psychology Review*, 26(8), 1041–1053.

Kershaw, K., Jolly, J., Bhabra, K. & Ford, J. (2005). Randomised controlled trial of community debriefing following operative delivery. *BJOG*, 112(11), 1504–1509.

Larkin, P., Begley, C. M. & Devane, D. (2009). Women's experiences of labour and birth: An evolutionary concept analysis. *Midwifery*, 25(2), e49–59.

Larsson, A.-K. & Dykes, A.-K. (2009). Care during pregnancy and childbirth in Sweden: Perspectives of Lesbian Women. *Midwifery*, 25(6), 682–690.

Lavender, T. & Walkinshaw, S. A. (1998). Can midwives reduce postpartum psychological morbidity? A randomized trial. *Birth (Berkeley, Calif.)*, 25(4), 215–219.

Lavender, T., Walkinshaw, S. A. & Walton, I. (1999). A prospective study of women's views of factors contributing to a positive birth experience. Midwifery, 15(1), 40–46.

Li, Y., Long, Z., Cao, D. & Cao, F. (2017). Social support and depression across the perinatal period: A longitudinal study. *J. Clin. Nurs.*, 26(17–18), 2776–2783.

Lindberg, I. & Engström, Å. (2013). A qualitative study of new fathers' experiences of care in relation to complicated childbirth. *Sexual & Reproductive Healthcare*, 4(4), 147–152.

Longworth, M. K., Furber, C. & Kirk, S. (2015). A narrative review of fathers' involvement during labour and birth and their influence on decision making. *Midwifery*, 31(9), 844–857.

Longworth, H. L. & Kingdon, C. K. (2011). Fathers in the birth room: What are they expecting and experiencing? A phenomenological study. *Midwifery*, 27(5), 588–594.

Lundgren, I., Andrén, K., Nissen, E. & Berg, M. (2013). Care seeking during the latent phase of labour – frequencies and birth outcomes in two delivery wards in Sweden. *Sexual and Reproductive Healthcare*, 4(4), 141–146.

Marrs, C., Ferarro, D., Cross, C. & McMurray, J. (2013). Understanding maternal cognitive changes: Associations between hormones and memory. *Hormones Matter*, 1–13.

McKenzie-Mcharg, K., Ayers, S., Ford, E., Horsch, A., Jomeen, J., Sawyer, A., Stramrood, C., Thomson, G. & Slade, P. (2015). Post-traumatic stress disorder following childbirth: An update of current issues and recommendations for future research. *Journal of Reproductive and Infant Psychology*, 1–19.

McManus, A. J., Hunter, L. P. & Renn, H. (2006). Lesbian experiences and needs during childbirth: Guidance for health care providers. *Journal of Obstetric, Gynecologic, and Neonatal Nursing*, 35(1), 13–23.

McNeill, J., Doran, J., Lynn, F., Anderson, G. & Alderdice, F. (2012). Public health education for midwives and midwifery students: a mixed methods study. *BMC Pregnancy and Childbirth*, 12(1), 142–142.

McNiven, P. S., Williams, J. I., Hodnett, E., Kaufman, K. & Hannah, M. E. (1998). An early labor assessment program: A randomized, controlled trial. *Birth*, 25(1), 5–10.

Meades, R., Pond, C., Ayers, S. & Warren, F. (2011). Postnatal debriefing: Have we thrown the baby out with the bath water? *Behav Res Ther*, 49(5), 367–372.

Miller, W. & Rollnick, S. (2004). Talking oneself into change: Motivational interviewing, stages of change, and therapeutic process. *Journal of Cognitive Psychotherapy*, 18(4), 299–308.

Murphy, D. J., Pope, C., Frost, J. & Liebling, R. E. (2003). Women's views on the impact of operative delivery in the second stage of labour: Qualitative interview study. *British Medical Journal*, 327(7424), 1132–1135.

Murray, L., Halligan, S. L. & Cooper, P. J. (2010). Effects of postnatal depression on mother-infant interactions, and child development. In G. Bremner, & T. Wachs (eds), *Handbook of infant development*. Chichester, UK: Wiley-Blackwell.

NHS England (2019). *NHS Long Term Plan.* London: NHS England. Available online: www.longtermplan.nhs.uk/wp-content/uploads/2019/01/nhs-long-term-plan-june-2019.pdf [Accessed June 17 2019].

NICE (2007). *Antenatal and postnatal mental health.* London: The British Psychological Society and The Royal College of Psychiatrists.

O'Gara, G. & Pattison, N. (2016). A qualitative exploration into the long-term perspectives of patients receiving critical care diaries across the United Kingdom. *Intensive and Critical Care Nursing*, 36, 1–7.

Peeler, S., Chung, M. C., Stedmon, J. & Skirton, H. (2013). A review assessing the current treatment strategies for postnatal psychological morbidity with a focus on post-traumatic stress disorder. *Midwifery*, 29(4), 377–388.

Poole, H., Mason, L. & Osborn, T. (2006). Women's views of being screened for postnatal depression. *Community Practitioner*, 79(11), 363–367.

Premberg, Å., Carlsson, G., Hellström, A.-L. & Berg, M. (2011). First-time fathers' experiences of childbirth—A phenomenological study. *Midwifery*, 27(6), 848–853.

Priest, S., Henderson, J., Evans, S. & Hagan, R. (2003). Stress debriefing after childbirth: randomised controlled trial. *MJA*, 178, 542–545.

RCOG (2011). *Operative Vaginal Delivery – Green-top Guideline No. 26.* London: ROCG.

RCOG (2015). *Blood Transfusion in Obstetrics. Green-top Guideline No. 47.* London: Royal College of Obstetricians and Gynaecologists.

RCOG (2017). Prevention and management of postpartum haemorrhage. Green-Top Guideline No. 52. *BJOG: An International Journal of Obstetrics and Gynaecology*, 124(5), e106–e149.

Riggs, D. S., Rothbaum, B. O. & Foa, E. B. (1995). A prospective examination of symptoms of post-traumatic stress disorder in victims of nonsexual assault. *Journal of Interpersonal Violence*, 10(2), 201–214.

Roberts, N. P., Kitchiner, N. J., Kenardy, J. & Bisson, J. I. (2009). Multiple session early psychological interventions for the prevention of post-traumatic stress disorder. *Cochrane Database of Systematic Reviews* (3).

Rose, S. C., Bisson, J., Churchill, R. & Wessely, S. (2002). Psychological debriefing for preventing post traumatic stress disorder (PTSD). *Cochrane Database of Systematic Reviews* (2).

Ryding, E., Wiren, E., Johansson, G., Ceder, B. & Dahlstrom, A. (2004). Group counseling for mothers after emergency cesarean section: A randomized controlled trial of intervention. *Birth*, 31(4), 247–253.

Seng, S. J., Low, K. L., Sperlich, L. M., Ronis, L. D. & Liberzon, L. I. (2009). Prevalence, trauma history, and risk for posttraumatic stress disorder among nulliparous women in maternity care. *Obstetrics and Gynecology*, 114(4), 839–847.

Shalev, A. Y., Gevonden, M., Ratanatharathorn, A., Laska, E., van Der Mei, W. F., Qi, W., Lowe, S., Lai, B. S., Bryant, R. A., Delahanty, D., Matsuoka, Y. J., Olff, M., Schnyder, U., Seedat, S., Deroon-Cassini, T. A., Kessler, R. C. & Koenen, K. C. (2019). Estimating the risk of PTSD in recent trauma survivors: Results of the International Consortium to Predict PTSD (ICPP). *World Psychiatry: Official Journal of the World Psychiatric Association (WPA)*, 18(1), 77–87.

Sheen, K. & Slade, P. (2015). The efficacy of 'debriefing' after childbirth: Is there a case for targeted intervention? *Journal of Reproductive and Infant Psychology*, 33(3), 308–320.

Skibniewski-Woods, D. (2011). A review of postnatal debriefing of mothers following traumatic delivery. *Community Practitioner*, 84(12), 29–32.

Small, R., Lumley, J., Donohue, L., Potter, A. & Waldenström, U. (2000). Randomised controlled trial of midwife led debriefing to reduce maternal depression after operative childbirth. *BMJ: British Medical Journal*, 321(7268), 1043–1047.

Steen, M., Downe, S., Bamford, N. & Edozien, L. (2011). Not-patient and not-visitor: A metasynthesis fathers' encounters with pregnancy, birth and maternity care. *Midwifery*, 28(4), 362–371.

Stein, A., Pearson, R., Goodman, S., Rapa, E., Rahman, A., McCallum, M., Howard, L. & Pariante, C. (2014). Effects of perinatal mental disorders on the fetus and child. *The Lancet*, 384(9956), 1800–1819.

Storksen, H. T., Garthus-Niegel, S., Vangen, S. & Eberhard-Gran, M. (2013). The impact of previous birth experiences on maternal fear of childbirth. *Acta Obstetricia Et Gynecologica Scandinavica*, 92(3), 318–324.

Stott, R. (2007). When head and heart do not agree: A theoretical and clinical analysis of rational-emotional dissociation (RED) in cognitive therapy. *Journal of cognitive Psychotherapy*, 21(1), 37–50.

Thomson, G. & Garrett, C. (2019). Afterbirth support provision for women following a traumatic/distressing birth: Survey of NHS hospital trusts in England. *Midwifery*, 71, 63–70.

Touqmatchi, D., Schwaiger, N. & Cotzias, C. (2011). How good are obstetric and gynaecology trainees at reviewing and debriefing their patients following operative deliveries? *Journal of Obstetrics and Gynaecology*, 31(8), 687–691.

Vallin, E., Nestander, H. & Wells, M. B. (2019). A literature review and meta-ethnography of fathers' psychological health and received social support during unpredictable complicated childbirths. *Midwifery*, 68, 48–55.

Waldenstrom, U., Hildingsson, I., Rubertsson, C. & Radestad, I. (2004). A negative birth experience: Prevalence and risk factors in a national sample. *Birth-Issues in Perinatal Care*, 31(1), 17–27.

Watkins, P. (2001). *Mental health nursing: The art of compassionate care*. Oxford: Butterworth-Heinemann.

Williams, C., Patricia Taylor, E. & Schwannauer, M. (2016). A Web-based survey of mother-infant bond, attachment experiences, and metacognition in posttraumatic stress following childbirth. *Infant Ment Health J*, 37(3), 259–273.

5 Therapeutic interventions

The next step

Introduction

Many women with perinatal mental illness (PMI) will not seek help in the postnatal period. This is often attributed to a sense of stigma and being seen as a 'bad mother', described as an external stigma or because they themselves (internal stigma) feel inferior and unable to meet society's expectation of a 'good mother' (see Chapter 1) (Button et al, 2017). Women also fear losing custody of their children (Millett et al, 2018). In addition, specialist services are patchy with approximately half of women with PMI not being identified or treated (Bauer et al, 2014). Whilst it is hoped that investment and expansion will follow with the ambitions outlined in the NHS Long Term Plan (NHS England, 2019), this will take time. When a woman does present and discloses how she feels, it is important that we acknowledge and have the knowledge and confidence to signpost to the appropriate available services. For anxiety and depression postpartum, this is likely to be primary health services. However, if the woman presents with signs of post-traumatic stress disorder (PTSD), services locally may be more limited. When we provide women with a service such as birth afterthoughts, women will present with PTSD. It is important that as part of this service there is a referral pathway for appropriate support and treatment.

Accessing psychological therapies postpartum

The majority of women that we see through a birth afterthoughts service will not require further input from perinatal mental health services and/or more specifically from a specialist psychology service. As discussed in Chapter 4, post-traumatic stress disorder (PTSD) is not normally diagnosed until at least four weeks following trauma and we recommend seeing women in birth afterthoughts after six weeks. Any signposting or referral at this point to PNMH or to a specialist psychology service like a birth trauma clinic, are likely to be appropriate referrals.

To address the need for greater access to NICE recommended psychological therapies for depression and anxiety disorders in the general population the Improving Access to Psychological Therapies (IAPT) programme has existed since 2007, predominantly with treatment based on cognitive behavioural therapy (CBT) principles (Clark, 2011). Further recommendations have stipulated that support should be tailored to the perinatal context (Department of Health, 2013). Despite this, there is criticism that much of what is offered by IAPT is still too prescriptive and not tailored to the needs of postpartum women with little opportunity to explore associated issues such as relationship issues post-birth, and women finding it process driven and impersonal (Millett et al, 2018). It is important to remember that IAPT services predominately work with mild to moderate anxiety and depression in the general population. For the treatment of PTSD relating specifically to birth trauma, it is unlikely that the provision of services available locally through IAPT would be able to provide the type of specialist support and treatment required.

In our experience, a Birth Trauma service should be delivered collaboratively with both maternity and psychology services working together to deliver a stepped care model. That may be with psychologists working within PNMH networks or delivered as part of the wider remit of psychological services within a hospital NHS Trust. Services can be funded through specialist commissioning arrangements or directly by the obstetric directorate within an NHS Trust. If women are seen first through a birth afterthoughts service after six weeks postnatal and appropriately screened for PTSD, the numbers of women requiring treatment are small (Brodrick et al, 2018). Investing in postpartum mental health will bring benefits not only to women and families, but also in the longer term to society, with the benefits of intervention sufficient to justify the additional spending (Bauer et al, 2014). In addition, if left untreated and women return in a subsequent pregnancy, unresolved psychological morbidity, such as maternal stress and more specifically psycho-traumatic stress from unresolved PTSD, is linked to negative outcomes for mother and fetus including pre-term birth (Kramer et al, 2009; Seng et al, 2011) and maternal request caesarean section (Ryding et al, 2015) (see Chapter 6), both of which have financial implications for obstetric services.

Providing a birth trauma service

From our experience, providing a service 'in-house' ensures close collaboration between both psychology services and maternity, allowing for a more seamless referral pathway and joined-up working, and providing women with more efficient and comprehensive care. It also ensures that each discipline informs the other. Midwives working in the birth afterthoughts service and the birth trauma clinical psychologists can discuss referrals and seek consultation from one another where appropriate: midwives may, for example, discuss appropriate referral routes with the psychologist, and the psychologist may, for example, seek advice regarding the obstetric details of a woman's experience or to understand whether a woman's perception of 'life threatening' is a true appraisal.

When women attend the Birth Trauma clinic, they are seen by a clinical psychologist who carries out a psychological assessment over one or two sessions. This consists of a clinical interview looking into what the woman's experience is in the here and now. The initial assessment does not focus on the events of the birth, but rather, how the woman is feeling about the birth, and how her memories of the birth, and other PTSD symptoms, are impacting on her now. A central part of the initial assessment is also consideration of the woman's life history prior to the birth, including her experience of the pregnancy, other reproductive events in her life, her significant relationships, any previous mental health difficulties, and other important events she has experienced, going back to her childhood and relevant family history. While that list may sound extensive, it is by no means exclusive, and the assessment may cover a myriad of other factors, depending on the woman's history and presentation. The assessment will also focus on how she has been responding to her distress and managing her feelings about the birth to get a sense of her coping style, and how this may be a helpful or maintaining factor in the presentation of her symptoms. There will be careful attention paid to the woman's strengths as well as her vulnerabilities. The psychologist uses all of this information to construct with the woman a 'formulation' of her experiences, which is a way of bringing all of these different factors together within the framework of a psychological model to essentially tell the woman's story. A formulation is a way of describing what has happened for the woman, and what is happening for her now. The formulation then informs what type of intervention is offered, and how this is applied.

It is imperative that psychological interventions are formulation driven, rather than delivered according to diagnosis. A diagnosis is usually the product of an expert making a judgement about the nature and severity of a person's symptoms. While this is necessary and helpful in most health-related scenarios, it can be a problematic approach in psychological therapy. Two women, for example, may both present with symptoms fulfilling diagnostic criteria for PTSD, but these may be expressed in very different ways. Understanding the individual experience and using this to inform intervention therefore avoids a reductionist 'one size fits all model' that would leave many women's psychological needs unmet.

Women are typically offered two assessment sessions and up to six treatment sessions, although this may be increased or reduced according to the woman's needs. Sessions last up to ninety minutes, as recommended for trauma-focused work (Grey, 2007). Women are usually seen in the antenatal clinic area of the maternity unit of the hospital. This choice of location has a dual function in that it allows for better integration of the psychology service into the maternity service, but it also begins to facilitate the therapeutic process of women's exposure to trauma-related stimuli. For some women, their avoidance symptoms are such that attending sessions in the maternity unit would become a barrier to them accessing a much-needed therapeutic intervention. In these cases, provision is made to see the women elsewhere in the hospital.

Therapeutic approaches

The psychological interventions offered within a Birth Trauma clinic should be consistent with relevant guidelines from the National Institute for Health and Care Excellence (NICE). These include guidelines for antenatal and postnatal mental health (NICE, 2014) which recommend that support and treatment should be offered after a traumatic birth, in line with NICE's recommendations on PTSD (NICE, 2018). In both guidelines, NICE specify the use of a high-intensity psychological intervention, namely eye movement desensitisation and reprocessing (EMDR) or trauma-focused cognitive behaviour therapy (CBT).

Eye movement desensitisation and reprocessing

EMDR is a short-term psychotherapeutic model developed in the 1980s (Shapiro, 1989). Traditionally, it involves a standardised protocol in which a thorough assessment is first carried out, followed by the development of a clear formulation. Next, the woman is trained in emotional regulation skills in order to manage the feelings arising from processing distressing memories. Following the establishment of such skills, further details are gained about the specific 'target memory' and the accompanying cognitions and bodily sensations. This memory is then 'processed' using a procedure whereby the woman is guided to recall the worst aspect of the memory whilst simultaneously being directed to engage in 'bilateral stimulation', usually moving their eyes from side to side. It is thought that this allows the brain to access the dysfunctionally encoded aspects of the memory and stimulate the processing systems to bring the memories to an adaptive resolution (for a summary of EMDR and its theoretical underpinnings, see Logie, 2014). Although there is a strong evidence base for the use of EMDR in treating PTSD, there is much less evidence about its use in treating PTSD after childbirth, with a particular lack of controlled studies (Baas et al, 2017).

Trauma-focused CBT

CBT has become widely applied across the country because of its strong evidence base across a wide range of psychological problems (for a meta-analysis, see Hofmann et al, 2012). This includes PTSD, with therapeutic interventions based on cognitive models such as that by Ehlers and Clark (2000), resulting in large effect sizes (for example, see Ehlers et al, 2005). Grey (2007) explains the aims of trauma-focused CBT deriving from the Ehlers and Clark (2000) model as including the reduction of re-experiencing symptoms via elaboration of the trauma memory, discrimination of memory triggers and integration of the memory into the autobiographical memory base, addressing negative appraisals of the trauma and its consequences, and change the maintaining factors of numbing and avoidance which are understandable coping strategies but preventing processing and reappraisal to take place. This is achieved through a variety of techniques, including psycho-education about the impact of trauma, and reliving the trauma memories whilst engaging in a process of 'cognitive restructuring', particularly of the 'hot spots' within the trauma memory. Grey (2007) also emphasises the importance of the therapeutic relationship, where the therapist provides both a physically and psychologically safe environment. In addition to the wide and robust evidence base for CBT as a treatment for PTSD mentioned previously, there is some evidence that it can be successfully applied to PTSD following childbirth (for example, see Ayers et al, 2007), although again, this is more limited.

Compassion-focused therapy

Compassion-focused therapy (CFT) was developed by Paul Gilbert (2000) within the context of a 'growing global movement' emphasising the transformative potential of compassion in a range of sectors, including business, education and health (Leaviss & Uttley, 2015). Based on attachment and evolutionary theory, Gilbert (2000) noted that much psychopathology is driven by high levels of shame and self-criticism. CFT was therefore developed to address this, by helping individuals to learn self-soothing techniques and create a more affiliative relationship with themselves and others (Beaumont & Hollins Martin, 2015). It has been noted that while fear is generally thought to be the dominant emotion in PTSD, for many people, shame and guilt is also central. Michelle Cree (2015) explains how this can affect mothers in that when our brains generate certain emotional responses, such as anxiety, anger, difficult intrusive thoughts and ideas, or a sense of disconnection from our baby, we can believe that we should not feel that way, and these emotions can then lead to a sense of shame. Trauma can be associated with shame in several ways. People who have experienced trauma can feel shame in relation to the event itself, and for how they respond afterwards: 'We can feel ashamed about who we are, what we have been through, what it makes us feel like inside and what we believe other people will now think of us if they knew what had happened' (Lee, 2012, p. 75).

Gilbert (2009) explains that CFT is influenced by research into the neurophysiology of emotion, which proposes three distinct emotional regulation systems: threat and protection systems; drive, resource seeking and excitement systems; and contentment, soothing and safeness systems. It is suggested that these systems have evolved to meet a range of survival needs in humans and other mammals, but can become unbalanced through lived experience. The experience of trauma, for example, heightens the threat system, resulting in an overdeveloped awareness of danger, which leads people to lack a sense of safety within themselves and their interpersonal relationships. The contentment/soothing system may become less accessible, particularly if this system was under-stimulated in a person's early life. CFT therefore focuses on activating the soothing system by introducing attributes and skills of compassion (Gilbert, 2009). Lee (2012) refers to the 'compassionate mind' as the 'antidote' to the 'threat-focused mind'.

CFT is considered a 'third-wave' cognitive therapy, and its use is therefore compliant with NICE guidelines for PTSD. There is evidence for its successful integration with CBT in the treatment of PTSD (Beaumont & Hollins Martin, 2015). In our experience, it is widely applicable to the women seen within the Birth Trauma clinic, who often present with high levels of shame and self-criticism relating to the birth experience (for example, 'my body failed'), and to their subsequent feelings (for example, 'I'm a terrible mother for feeling this way').

Measuring effectiveness of psychology informed interventions

In the service we offer women attending the Birth Trauma service are asked to complete a set of standardised outcome measures at assessment, and again at the end of their intervention. These measures help to inform the clinical assessment and formulation, and also give an indication of clinical change. To capture the range of psychological distress a woman may be experiencing, the data set currently consists of the PHQ-9 measure of depression (Kroenke et al, 2001) and the GAD-7 measure of anxiety (Spitzer et al, 2006). The PHQ-9 and GAD-7 are widely used in mental health services. The most specific outcome measure is the Impact of Event Scale, revised version (IES-R, Weiss & Marmar, 1996), a self-report measure consisting of three subscales reflecting the PTSD diagnostic domains of intrusion, avoidance and hyperarousal. An evaluation of the data routinely collected in the clinic during its first seven years of operation confirmed that women experience significant reductions in scores on all measures of anxiety symptoms (Brodrick et al, 2018). Average total scores on the IES-R measure of PTSD symptoms fell from above to below the clinical cut-off, and general levels of anxiety were also reduced. For women seen postnatally, depression scores were also significantly lower post-intervention than at assessment. Women who were seen for treatment in a subsequent pregnancy did not experience a significant reduction in depression symptoms, but had generally lower depressive symptoms at assessment anyway. This preliminary analysis shows that the Birth Trauma clinic provides effective short-term psychological treatment for women experiencing symptoms of PTSD following childbirth.

Moving forward

Within the remit of psychological trauma post-partum the Birth Trauma clinic is currently a relatively small service specifically for women with PTSD following childbirth. Wider access and integration of psychology services locally, regionally and nationally, if the NHS Long-term Plan (2019) is to be realised, is much needed to increase the provision of appropriate informed psychological therapies to women postpartum. In addition there is a need to include access for partners who also experience distress and depression post-birth and are at risk of psychological morbidity including PTSD (Hinton et al, 2014), as discussed in Chapter 4. As maternity services continue to work towards more family inclusive services

(NHS England, 2016) with fathers/partners seen as integral to the mother–infant dyad, we must ensure they too have access to appropriate mental health services and support.

In addition if local maternity services have integrated psychology services it would allow for a more systemic trauma-informed service model to be implemented, in which further work is done with midwives, health visitors and GPs to support them in recognising psychological distress in women after childbirth, and how best to respond. We know that many women will experience distress after childbirth, but only a small proportion of these will need specialist support to recover. The majority, however, would benefit from compassionate, supportive listening and care from their natural circle of support, including the professionals who play such a key role in routine post-partum care.

Conclusion

Whilst not all localities will have access to a Birth Trauma clinic, it is important that all maternity staff are aware of the services offered locally for women and partners with birth trauma as well as local support groups and online groups which it appears women find useful for gaining a shared understanding and discourse with other mothers experiencing PMI (Moore & Ayers, 2016). Psychological interventions for birth trauma must be formulation driven, understanding the uniqueness of each women and what has shaped her experience rather than a diagnosis driven generic therapeutic intervention. As PMI receives continued political investment and interest it is hoped that access and availability of psychology informed interventions postpartum will become equitable across all regions, alongside an expansion of new and existing services.

References

Ayers, S., McKenzie-Mcharg, K. & Eagle, A. (2007). Cognitive behaviour therapy for postnatal post-traumatic stress disorder: Case studies. *Journal of Psychosomatic Obstetrics and Gynecology*, 28(3), 177–184.

Baas, M. A. M., Stramrood, C. A. I., Dijksman, L. M., De Jongh, A. & Van Pampus, M. G. (2017). The OptiMUM-study: EMDR therapy in pregnant women with posttraumatic stress disorder after previous childbirth and pregnant women with fear of childbirth: design of a multicentre randomized controlled trial. *European Journal of Psychotraumatology*, 8(1).

Bauer, A., Parsonage, M., Knapp, M., Lemmi, V. & Adelaja, B. (2014). The costs of perinatal mental health problems. *Centre for Mental Health and LSE.*

Beaumont, E. & Hollins Martin, C. (2015). A narrative review exploring the effectiveness of Compassion-Focused Therapy. *Counselling Psychology Review*, 30(1), 21–32.

Brodrick, A., Slade, P., Saradjian, A., Williamson, E. & Pipeva, A. (2018). The Birth Trauma Psychological Therapy Service: A stepped care service model. [Poster] Royal College of Midwifery Annual Conference. Manchester.

Button, S., Thornton, A., Lee, S., Shakespeare, J. & Ayers, S. (2017). Seeking help for perinatal psychological distress: A meta-synthesis of women's experiences. *The British Journal of GeneralPpractice: The Journal of the Royal College of General Practitioners*, 67(663), e692–e699.

Clark, D. M. (2011). Implementing NICE guidelines for the psychological treatment of depression and anxiety disorders: The IAPT experience. *International Review of Psychiatry*, 23(4), 318–327.

Cree, M. (2015). *Postnatal depression: Using compassion focused therapy to enhance mood, confidence and bonding.* London: Robinson.

Department of Health (2013). *IAPT Perinatal Positive Practice Guide.* London: Department of Health,. Available online: www.uea.ac.uk/documents/246046/11919343/perinatal-positive-practice-guide-2013.pdf/ [Accessed 25 July 2019].

Ehlers, A. & Clark, D. M. (2000). A cognitive model of posttraumatic stress disorder. *Behaviour Research and Therapy*, 38(4), 319–345.

Ehlers, A., Clark, D. M., Hackmann, A., McManus, F. & Fennell, M. (2005). Cognitive therapy for post-traumatic stress disorder: Development and evaluation. *Behaviour Research and Therapy*, 43(4), 413–431.

Gilbert, P. (2000). The relationship of shame, social anxiety and depression: The role of the evaluation of social rank. *Clinical Psychology and Psychotherapy*, 7(3), 174–189.

Gilbert, P. (2009). Introducing compassion-focused therapy. *Advances in Psychiatric Treatment*, 15(3), 199–208.

Grey, N. (2007). Posttraumatic stress disorder: Treatment. In S. Lindsay & G. Powell, (eds), *The handbook of clinical adult psychology.* London: Routledge.

Hinton, L., Locock, L. & Knight, M. (2014). Partner experiences of "near-miss" events in pregnancy and childbirth in the UK: A qualitative study. *PLoS One*, 9(4), e91735.

Hofmann, S., Asnaani, A., Vonk, I., Sawyer, A. & Fang, A. (2012). The efficacy of cognitive behavioral therapy: A review of meta-analyses. *Cognitive Therapy and Research*, 36(5), 427–440.

Kramer, M. S., Lydon, J., Seguin, L., Goulet, L., Kahn, S. R. & McNamara, H. (2009). Stress pathways to spontaneous preterm birth: The role of stressors, psychological distress, and stress hormones. *Am J Epidemiology*, 169(1319–1326).

Kroenke, K., Spitzer, R. L. & Williams, J. B. (2001). The PHQ-9: Validity of a brief depression severity measure. *Journal of General Internal Medicine*, 16(9), 606–616.

Leaviss, J. & Uttley, L. (2015). Psychotherapeutic benefits of compassion-focused therapy: An early systematic review, *Psychological Medicine*, 45(5), 927–945.

Lee, D. (2012). *Recovering from trauma using compassion focused therapy*. London: Robinson.

Logie, R. (2014). EMDR – more than just a therapy for PTSD? *The Psychologist*, 27, 512–517.

Millett, L., Howard, L., Bick, D., Stanley, N. & Johnson, S. (2018). Experiences of improving access to psychological therapy services for perinatal mental health difficulties: A qualitative study of women's and therapists' views. *Behavioural and Cognitive Psychotherapy*, 46(4), 421–436.

Moore, D. & Ayers, S. (2016). Virtual voices: social support and stigma in postnatal mental illness Internet forums. *Psychology, Health and Medicine*, 1–6.

NICE (2014). *Antenatal and postnatal mental health: Clinical management and service guidance CG192.* London: National Institute for Health and Care Excellence. Available online: www.nice.org.uk/guidance/cg192/resources/antenatal-and-postnatal-mental-health-clinical-management-and-service-guidance-pdf-35109869806789 [Accessed 4 November 2019]

NICE (2018). *Post traumatic stress disorder: Management (CG116).* London: National Institute for Health and Care Excellence.

NHS England (2016) *Better Births: Improving outcomes of maternity services in England – a five year forward view for maternity care.* London: NHS England. Available online: www.england.nhs.uk/wp-content/uploads/2016/02/national-maternity-review-report.pdf [Accessed 1 July 2019].

NHS England (2019). *NHS Long Term Plan.* London: NHS England. Available online: www.longtermplan.nhs.uk/wp-content/uploads/2019/01/nhs-long-term-plan-june-2019.pdf [Accessed 17 June 2019].

Ryding, E. L., Lukasse, M., van Parys, A., Wangel, A., Karro, H., H., K., Schroll, A. & Schei, B. (2015). Fear of childbirth and risk of cesarean delivery: A cohort study in six European countries. *Birth*, 42(1), 48–55.

Seng, J., Low, L., Sperlich, M., Ronis, D. & Liberzon, I. (2011). Post-traumatic stress disorder, child abuse history, birthweight and gestational age: A prospective cohort study. *BJOG: An International Journal of Obstetrics and Gynaecology*, 118(11), 1329–1339.

Shapiro, F. (1989). Efficacy of the eye movement desensitization procedure in the treatment of traumatic memories. *Journal of Traumatic Stress*, 2(2), 199–223.

Spitzer, R. L., Kroenke, K., Williams, J. B. W. & Löwe, B. (2006). A brief measure for assessing generalized anxiety disorder: The GAD-7. *Archives of Internal Medicine*, 166(10), 1092–1097.

Weiss, D. S. & Marmar, C. R. (1996). The impact of event scale – Revised. In J. P. Wilson & T. M. Keane (eds), *Assessing psychological trauma and PTSD*. New York: Guilford Press.

6 Supporting women in their next pregnancy

Introduction

We introduced a birth afterthoughts service locally in 2011. The addition of a psychology pathway followed shortly after, and then, as a natural progression, an antenatal service provision for women who are anxious and/or fearful of birth. From experience, women who are seen in birth afterthoughts feel reassured when they understand they can access a similar service when they are next pregnant to re-open discussions and plan for care.

In Sweden, every maternity unit offers a midwife-led counselling service for women who are fearful of childbirth (Larsson et al, 2016). In the UK, although some maternity units do offer an additional service (Richens et al, 2015), there is no national guidance around assessment of childbirth-related anxiety or fear of childbirth and no mandated service provision. However, within the publication of the NHS Long-term Plan (NHS England, 2019) and acknowledgement of the financial burden of perinatal mental health (Bauer et al, 2014), there is now a commitment to establish evidence-based psychological support and therapy within perinatal mental health services and an understanding that provision of services needs to increase from pre-conception to twenty-four months post-birth. Irrespective of what is available locally, women will present with anxiety and fear in pregnancy, with concerns often voiced first to their community midwife. What women want from this interaction is non-judgemental listening and understanding from a professional who is genuinely interested (Staneva et al, 2015).

Understanding pregnancy-related anxiety

There is a general consensus that pregnancy is a stressful time for women with challenges to adapt to physical, psychosocial and psychological changes (Hodgkinson et al, 2014) and worries about the health of the baby which have been reported to be present in 76 per cent of pregnant women (DiPietro et al, 2009). Some degree of anxiety is therefore probably a normal aspect of pregnancy, and it has been suggested that it is a healthy indicator of women engaging in the motherhood task of protecting the fetus from harm (Harpel, 2008). However for some women, anxiety relating specifically to pregnancy and/or birth can become overwhelming and interfere with normal functioning and cognition. Distinct from generalised anxiety disorder (GAD) and depression states, this type of anxiety which is related specifically to the state of being pregnant, is termed 'pregnancy-related anxiety' and is considered a distinct phenomenon (McMahon et al, 2013). In women with GAD, the anxiety is likely to continue post-birth, whereas with pregnancy-related anxiety, it should diminish after birth (Huizink et al, 2014). Assessing for generalised anxiety is important and guidance in the UK recommends using the two-item Generalised Anxiety Disorder scale (NICE, 2014). Women tend to be signposted to their GP, or for locally delivered, low-intensity psychological interventions. The NICE guidance on Antenatal and Postnatal mental health (NICE, 2014) focuses on depression, anxiety disorders, eating disorders, drug and alcohol-use disorders and severe mental illness but does not discuss pregnancy-related anxiety. Tokophobia is mentioned once with advice to refer to a healthcare professional with expertise in perinatal mental health.

Pregnancy-related anxiety and fears tend to focus on areas such as health of the baby, appearance-related concerns (Huizink et al, 2014) and a fear of childbirth (Saisto & Halmesmaki, 2003; Storksen et al, 2012). Depending on severity, it can result in physical symptoms of palpations, nausea and vomiting, and is a frequent cause of insomnia (Bayrampour et al, 2016). The anxiety can feel debilitating and is complicated further by societal expectations that women should feel happy and willing to sacrifice their own wellbeing for that of the baby (Staneva & Wigginton, 2018). This can lead to women feeling isolated and inadequate as their lived experience does not meet cultural norms of the 'good mother' and result in women choosing to avoid dealing with their fears by not discussing or outwardly showing their anxiety as way of coping (Staneva et al, 2015). This has been termed 'self-silencing' with women experiencing powerlessness and a need to withdraw their true selves from intimate and social support (Jack & Ali, 2010).

A lot of academic interest around pregnancy-related anxiety has centred around the effect to the developing fetus of elevated maternal cortisol levels due to stress, though the exact mechanism on fetal programming is still debated (Cherak et al, 2018). Whatever the underlying physiology, pregnancy-related anxiety is consistently and independently associated with small for gestational age birthweights (Littleton et al, 2007) and spontaneous pre-term birth (Kramer et al, 2009). This linear association between pregnancy anxiety and prematurity is considered to have an effect size comparable to cigarette smoking (Dunkel Schetter & Tanner, 2012). In addition, there is evidence of adverse neurodevelopmental outcomes in children when maternal anxiety, stress and depression are diagnosed prenatally (Van den Bergh et al, 2005). In terms of cost to the NHS, the reported financial cost of maternal and child health as a result of pregnancy-related anxiety is £35,000 per case (Bauer et al, 2014)

Understanding fear of childbirth in the next pregnancy

When pregnancy-related anxiety is focused specifically on labour and birth, we start to use the term fear of childbirth (FOC) or tokophobia. However, we need to be careful how we apply these terms as there is no agreed measurement tool on which to base a diagnosis, and even when using the same measurement scale, different cut-off points have been used to define clinically significant fear (O'Connell et al, 2017). The origins of the term date back to the eighteenth century, when it was referred to as 'fear of parturition' by French psychiatrist Louis Victor Marce. This later became anglicised as 'fear of childbirth', defined as significantly affecting daily functioning and wellbeing (Nilsson et al, 2018). Tokophobia was originally defined within psychiatry as a 'pathological dread' and avoidance of childbirth (Hofberg & Ward, 2003), which can reach a specific phobia classification as defined by the *Diagnostic and Statistical Manual of Mental Disorders* (Wijma, 2003).

Whilst identifying heterogenous issues, the pooled prevalence of tokophobia worldwide is cited as 14 per cent, with good evidence that the rate has increased over the last thirty years (O'Connell et al, 2017). In another study, the same measurement scale was used across seven different European countries and rates of childbirth fear differed from 6.3 per cent in Belgium to 14.8 per cent in Estonia (Nilsson et al, 2018); this was similar to the study done by (Lukasse et al, 2014) with the same countries noted as being lower and higher and an overall incidence rate of 11 per cent. In Australia, rates have been reported as high as 23 per cent (O'Connell et al, 2017)

The link between previous negative birth experience, with and without symptoms of post-traumatic stress and a fear in subsequent pregnancies has been well proven and discussed (Dencker et al, 2019; Garthus-Niegel et al, 2011; Lukasse et al, 2014; Rouhe et al, 2009a; Saisto et al, 1999; Storksen et al, 2013). Whilst studies have cited obstetric complications such as emergency caesarean section as risk factors for fear in subsequent births (Rouhe et al, 2009a; Storksen et al, 2013), it is also acknowledged that if a woman feels safe and taken care of, then the overall experience can be positive despite complications (Garthus-Niegel et al, 2014). In a prospective study of parous women in Norway returning in a subsequent pregnancy, 80 per cent of study participants who had previous obstetric complications did not view the experience as negative and did not develop a fear of childbirth; fear was greatest in women with a previous subjective negative birth experience (Storksen et al, 2013). As discussed in Chapter 3, subjective elements including the attitudes of the staff delivering care and the perceived level of support in labour can have a huge impact on how a woman views her birth experience, and if perceived as missing from care, correlate with a negative birth experience (Fenwick et al, 2009; Fisher et al, 2006). (Sheen & Slade, 2018) describe three elements of women's fears:

1. physiological – fear of injury to self or infant, fear of pain, physical incapacity
2. psychological – fear of the unknown, loss of control, lack of emotional capacity
3. sociological – fear of poor care, inadequate support, professional competence

Whilst understanding these specific fears is important and as clinicians very relatable, if we want to support women, we also need an understanding of the underlying cognitive components that are ruminating through a woman's thought processes and, if not addressed, will continue to drive the anxiety.

Understanding the psychology behind fear

Fear of childbirth sits alongside the domain of anxiety to which it is interrelated and enables us to start to understand how it affects maternal behaviour. From personal experience, women often doubt their own ability and coping mechanisms when discussing fears 'I just know I won't be able to do that again'. This is often accompanied by an assertion of expected failure and/or of catastrophic harm occurring if they were to risk labouring again. These beliefs form part of the psychological make-up of the woman. This appraisal of labour and birth then forms the cognitive component of the anxiety and fear which consists of negative thoughts (Winton et al, 1995) and negative beliefs about oneself, the world or the future (Foa et al, 2006). This is often accompanied by a tendency to exaggerate negative aspects of future events (Beck, 1976) and a fear that one will lack personal mastery when exposed to a certain situation (i.e. childbirth), also referred to as self-efficacy (Bandura, 1997). People with a high sense of self-efficacy tend to visualise success, whereas those with low self-efficacy visualise failure and focus on things going wrong. Additionally, women with a FOC tend to have a perception that they will be unable to adapt and cope in a stressful situation (Soderquist et al, 2004).

When talking to women with a FOC, two other psychological phenomena frequently present, namely *intolerance of uncertainty* and *pain catastrophising*, both of which have shown to be positively predictive of fear of birth in pregnant women (Rondung et al, 2018).

An *intolerance of uncertainty* is associated extensively with anxiety disorders and is viewed as a transdiagnostic construct, meaning that it features across a number of mental health disorders including post-traumatic stress symptoms (Oglesby et al, 2016) as well as fear of childbirth (Sheen & Slade, 2018). Intolerance of uncertainty is conceptualised simply as how a person responds to uncertainties, with individuals feeling unable to endure the cognitive, emotional and/or behavioural responses that are triggered when outcomes are unknown or ambiguous (Dugas et al, 2005). This drives a behavioural response of avoidance as all uncertain events are interpreted as threatening (Carleton et al, 2007). In women with high levels of intolerance of uncertainty, it is easy to see why pregnancy and labour, which are by their very nature uncertain and unpredictable, are especially problematic.

Pain catastrophising is a negative cognitive-affective response to pain. Within the chronic pain literature, it is a well-known phenomenon, linked to the fear avoidance model whereby pain catastrophising and personal determinants, such as negative affectivity, affect how someone evaluates pain (Vlaeyen & Linton, 2000). Negative affectivity refers to a tendency by individuals to scan their environment for threat and interpret ambiguous stimuli in a negative and threatening manner. Pain catastrophising is typified by a predisposition to magnify the threat of pain and to feel helpless when anticipating a painful encounter, during the painful event and following a painful event (Quartana et al, 2009). In relation to childbirth, there is evidence that pain catastrophising is associated with higher ratings of both anticipated and experienced pain during childbirth (Flink et al, 2009; Junge et al, 2018) and a preference for choosing a planned caesarean section (Dehghani et al, 2014). We know that women fear intolerable pain during labour (Striebich et al, 2018). Understanding pain perception from a psychological perspective enables us to better understand how the anticipation of labour pain may be cognitively appraised by women during pregnancy.

These maladaptive cognitions strive to avoid the stress-inducing experience as a form of self-protection. This can manifest as 'safety behaviours' such as avoiding pregnancy, not continuing with a pregnancy (Zar et al, 2002) or requesting a planned caesarean section (Rouhe et al, 2009b). The anxiety is then maintained through an intricate thread of psychological responses feeding cognition and resultant avoidant safety behaviours. Engaging in such safety behaviours then prevents individuals from testing out the reality of their maladaptive cognitions, forming new, more adaptive cognitions and reducing their fear. This is why studies looking at women who request a planned CS due to fear find that they maintain levels of anxiety and fear despite having their choice of caesarean agreed and a date planned (Olieman et al, 2017).

In addition to the underlying psychological factors, the cultural context of birth in Western countries sees women exposed to a growing professional tolerance of rising CS rates and narratives that label vaginal birth as risky (Fenwick et al, 2006; Fenwick et al, 2010). In this way, there is a changing attitude amongst women towards accepting intervention in childbirth (Green & Baston, 2007). To women who are already fearful, this increased reliance on technology in labour and birth might be interpreted as transforming the unpredictable process of 'natural' childbirth to one that can be controlled (Fisher et al, 2006) and reinforce her own view that birth is risky and unwise.

Understanding this deeper causation, together with formulating why a woman feels the way she does, enables us to reflect and re-evaluate our own responses to women's fear, our attitudes to childbirth and our epistemological basis of what childbirth means. In this way, we can frame our responses in a way that is supportive, empathic and sensitive to the psychological and cultural implications of birth and motherhood which have already been explored in Chapter 1.

Assessing the fear of childbirth

Many of the validated scales for assessing FOC are suited more to research environments as culturally they can be difficult to translate and require time for completion and analysis (Richens et al, 2018). For ease of clinical application, the Fear of Birth Scale (Haines et al, 2011) provides good internal consistency and construct validity (Rondung et al, 2018). This is a simple tool consisting of two visual analogue scales and would be suitable for use in clinical practice (O'Connell et al, 2017; Richens et al, 2018). Using a screening tool at the booking appointment may initially yield higher rates, with the rate likely to fall as the pregnancy progresses (Kingdon et al, 2009) and the woman has time to evaluate her feelings around this subsequent pregnancy.

One simple assessment would be to ask women who are booking in their second or subsequent pregnancy 'were there elements of your last birth that you found upsetting or difficult?' or even simply 'how was your last birth experience?' This gives women permission to voice concerns. Often, women have sealed their previous birth experience away, and when they become pregnant again, these fears or concerns come back to the forefront. The fact that women are able to articulate the construct of worries and fears and to identify what is important to them (Ternstrom et al, 2016) gives weight to the argument that when a woman expresses a FOC and asks for support, this could in itself be used as a definition (Saisto & Halmesmaki, 2003). Similarly, a request for a CS due to FOC should foremost be interpreted as a sign that she is in need of help (Dweik & Sluijs, 2015). As discussed in Chapter 4, approaching this discussion with sensitive dialogue and empathic support is in itself likely to be therapeutic, and should not be underestimated.

Supporting women with fear of childbirth

There is some evidence that a counselling type intervention for pregnant women with fear is beneficial (Striebich et al, 2018). A systematic review of non-pharmacological prenatal interventions concluded that short interventions delivered by experienced maternity staff that explore the reasons for the fear and then help women develop strategies to cope are effective for women with pregnancy-related anxiety and fear of birth (Stoll et al, 2018). In Australia, telephone psycho-education sessions delivered by midwives were found to be effective (Toohill et al, 2014), with a follow-up study showing a reduction in caesarean section for fear and a preference for vaginal birth in future pregnancies (Fenwick et al, 2015). In the UK, a yoga-based intervention was found to reduce levels of fear (Newham et al, 2014). There is also considerable evidence and learning to be gained from Sweden who started implementing fear of child-birth clinics twenty-five years ago (Larsson et al, 2016). The clinics are run by labour ward midwives with involvement of obstetricians, and have been shown to be valued by women, and enable women to feel more positive about birth (Wulcan & Nilsson, 2019). There is also evidence that these types of counselling interventions, regardless of birth outcome, are viewed positively by women in the short term (Larsson et al, 2015) and longer term up to two–four years later (Nerum et al, 2006). The value of a team based or caseload midwifery model which enable continuity of carer and known support in labour is likely to be valuable to these women (Hildingsson et al, 2018), although in a follow-up study which looked at the addition of antenatal counselling alongside a team midwifery approach fear of birth decreased significantly over time for all women irrespective of whether they were cared for in labour by a known midwife or not (Hildingsson et al, 2019). Antenatal counselling interventions tend to involve a patient-centred approach, an approach already discussed in Chapter 3, with time to discuss events of the last birth, explore fears, challenge misconceptions, in the same way as described in Chapter 4, and then work on the premise of promoting coping skills.

Midwives may feel ill-equipped to deal with such discussions as well as the pressure of being time limited. Additionally, there will be specific characteristics unique to that woman which also filter her response to events for instance how she herself was parented, her level of self-efficacy and self-esteem. All of these will frame her perception of events. To a woman who fears repeating the same experience, a simple assertion that all will be well this time is unlikely to be helpful, as it is purely responding to what we believe is the cause of the anxiety. A woman who had a long first labour due to an occipito-posterior presentation, for instance, may be reassured by the knowledge that in a second labour the body labours differently and is more efficient, but if the same woman describes perceived failings of the staff as the cause of her fear, how do we rationalise the fear to give her reassurance?

To frame our responses, it is useful as health professionals to have an understanding of how events are recorded and experienced by women. The ABC model (Ellis, 1994) used within cognitive behaviour therapy (CBT) is a useful way to illustrate this point:

Activating event: midwife was felt to be unfriendly and unsupportive
Beliefs: I am not worthy of compassionate care, I am not important, staff are cruel and not to be trusted
Consequences (emotional and behaviours): I am vulnerable, I feel scared, I have no control – I will avoid this scenario again

This model illustrates how it is the *beliefs* that frame the emotional response to events. These beliefs can be explored in the same way as described in Chapter 3 utilising active listening skills. This can then facilitate her ability to work through the emotions associated with her previous birth and separate them from the coming birth. Successful management of these emotions is about processing stressful life events appropriately such that they do not have any lasting negative effects on everyday life (Rachman, 2001). Dialogue in these circumstances needs to concentrate on facilitating a woman's coping mechanisms rather than assurances that everything will be ok (Halvorsen et al, 2010). The ABC model has been used as part of a study intervention to enable primiparous women to cope with their childbirth fears (Uçar & Golbasi, 2018), it was delivered as part of an educational programme over six sessions with results showing a reduction in fears and higher satisfaction levels with birth when compared to the control group.

Women need to feel confident that they can deal with any eventuality, including perceived poor attitudes amongst staff. Additionally, women need to feel confident about controlling their anxiety (Saisto & Halmesmaki, 2003); this might involve thinking through coping mechanisms and identifying what is important for personal security and to maintain a sense of control (Meyer, 2013). Measures which help to promote resilience and psychological preparedness to be able to deal with an unpredictable journey are important and have the potential to increase levels of self-efficacy and lead to a better experience of birth (Salmela-Aro et al, 2012).

Importance of social support

The availability of adequate social support plays an important buffering role in minimising distress and increasing self-esteem (Staneva et al, 2015), and there is clear evidence that fear of childbirth is more prevalent in women with poor social support (Lukasse et al, 2014; Toohill et al, 2015). This includes social networks which enable women to ask female relatives and friends about their experiences as well as partner support. The positive effects of social support on positive health outcomes is well known, with evidence that it reduces psychological stress in response to negative events and can mitigate the experiences of pain (Brown et al, 2003; Hornstein & Eisenberger, 2017).

The emotional and physical support that will be provided by the father or birth partner is also important to consider. From experience of talking to couples, there tends to be a sense that they will behave differently this time. The term 'respectively challenge' was used by one husband as well as the realisation that 'we will do things differently this time' which seems to occur as part of a reflective process. The change in behaviour tends to be focused around asking more questions, seeking clarification and also asserting choice, all of which are important to fathers, as when lacking leave them feeling excluded and uncertain (Vallin et al, 2019). The discourses also centre around wanting more control and avoiding the feeling of 'being done to' which are equally important to how a woman appraises her birth (Green & Baston, 2003; Waldenstrom et al, 2004). Discussion around reflecting on past experiences, understanding what each other expects and what is important may help couples to emotionally prepare. In addition, fathers may need guidance and information on how to provide support physically, and also how they might raise questions on behalf of their partner. When fathers feel able to provide this type of support it can promote a more positive birth experience for both parents (Alio et al, 2011; Awad & Bühling, 2011). Discussion around how decision making will be enacted during labour is therefore an important consideration for couples (Longworth et al, 2015) and an important component of the birth planning. Understanding the extent of partner support and exploring how collaboratively they can support each other through labour birth is an important consideration.

Dealing with a request for a CS due to fear

There is considerable evidence that fear of childbirth is linked to maternal request CS (Ryding et al, 2015). The debate around caesarean section on maternal request still seems to divide healthcare professionals (Sharpe et al, 2015) and also the media with reports that women are either too posh to push or have a right to choose (Rustin, 2016). Women are often torn between wanting to avoid emotional pain and recognising that vaginal birth is optimal for both her and her baby (Halvorsen et al, 2010). When a woman has had a previous birth it is about understanding what that emotional pain means to the woman and supporting her to realise the potential psychological problems that have motivated her desire for a CS.

From experience, women often request a caesarean believing that it will prevent previous sequelae, for instance a retained placenta after a long induction of labour process, and an emotionally difficult postnatal journey and breastfeeding experience. From a clinician perspective, a planned CS is irrational as it will not necessarily prevent retained placental tissue, will incur additional risks and add a longer physical recovery period to the postnatal experience. So, to the clinician's rational brain, choosing X to avoid Y seems illogical. This can be understood from the theoretical framework of crisis reactions (Caplan, 1964) which distinguishes between what could be described as an appropriate level of apprehension towards an event and an irrational reaction that seems much stronger than the actualising event would suggest is needed.

The usual pathway within the NHS, regardless of whether a woman is low risk midwife led, or high risk, is for the woman to be referred to an obstetric clinic for discussion. In some units, this is then followed by a referral to a second obstetrician (NICE, 2011). National guidance (NICE, 2011) is clear that a CS should be allowed but only after an exploration of the fears and any appropriate perinatal mental health support has been explored. How this is delivered locally is currently a postcode lottery with only 26 per cent of NHS Trusts fully compliant with NICE guidance (Birthrights, 2018).

In many NHS Trusts, there is not a pathway in place for women to discuss fears with someone trained in perinatal metal health, and it is unrealistic to expect an obstetrician in a busy antenatal clinic to explore in depth the woman's underlying beliefs, emotions and accompanying fear that has led to a request for a CS. The obstetricians role is to assess the clinical picture and ensure women are informed of the risks and benefits of a caesarean compared to a vaginal birth (NICE, 2011). In this way, the request for a CS is met with professional argument which stresses the physical risks involved in a CS but which adds little value (Nama & Wilcock, 2011) and is rated negatively by women (Karlstrom et al, 2011). It also ultimately, communicates to the woman that although a vaginal birth is recommended, it is ultimately her choice (Bryant et al, 2007). This autonomy-focused style of the dialogue is unhelpful on a number of levels:

1. How women view risks and how clinicians view risk are very different with women often more accepting of risk (Turner et al, 2008).
2. It does not acknowledge that the experience of childbirth is equally important to women and often juxtaposed towards a clinician view of what is medically best.
3. Without challenging her thought processes and asserting our professional confidence in her ability to physically and emotionally cope with labour again, we may send a message to the woman that she is right in believing she is unable to labour again.
4. It is delivered from the viewpoint that the woman desires a CS when it should be exploring why she doesn't want to consider vaginal birth.
5. Regardless of chosen mode of birth, psychological difficulties pertaining to the first birth experience remained unresolved.

In a study exploring differing counselling techniques utilised in a FOC clinic (Halvorsen et al, 2010), whilst both midwives used a patient-orientated approach to counsel the women, one midwife employed a 'coping attitude' approach and communicated ways in which the women could be helped to give birth vaginally, but the other used an 'autonomy attitude', which stressed that whilst vaginal is preferable, it is ultimately the woman's choice. The women who were counselled using a coping style were more likely to choose and achieve vaginal birth. The study also revealed that adopting a coping style can be easily learned through observation and critical reflection. Another way to frame discussions around maternal choice caesarean is to adopt some of the skills used in motivational interviewing, in particular the guiding style (Rollnick et al, 2008). Clinical discussions are often directing: 'having major abdominal surgery for no reason carries serious risks for you and your baby so we recommend vaginal birth'. From discussions with women and clinicians, this type of closed questioning on first meeting often leaves women feeling defensive, with the clinician in control and 'holding all the cards'. A guiding style using open questions and active listening would reset the discourse: 'from my side it is concerning that for a young healthy woman a caesarean can have significant health implications now and, in the future … but can you tell me what concerns you first …?' In this way, the clinician has handed control back to the woman and opened up a discussion.

From experience, a request for a CS is rarely a simple assertion by a woman to choose a CS as the preferred mode of birth option. It is more likely to be an assertion that she wants to minimise the potential of repeating the emotional journey of her previous birth and any psychological distress that she attributes to this previous birth. Therefore, conversations need to focus on coping and enabling rather than polar versions of vaginal versus caesarean birth. This is why, as is the case in Sweden where FOC clinics are well established, it is midwives who are best placed to support women (Larsson et al, 2016).

The ABC example above was framed around the sociological elements of birth experience. Using the example discussed above of a woman with a previous retained placenta wanting a CS it is easier to start to understand that the activating event is not as simple as an unexpected obstetric intervention or complications. Adopting a coping attitude, the model continues with the addition of D and E.

A: retained placenta-separation from baby immediately after birth; isolated from partner; partner distressed and left alone with newborn; breastfeeding difficult to establish.

B: my body failed to perform like it should; I failed my partner; my partner's distress is my fault; my baby suffered because I couldn't feed her; I am a bad mother.

C: it's best that I don't put us through that again; I am not cut out to give birth.

As discussed in Chapter 2, the 'beliefs' are magnified by societal expectations of women and motherhood. Often there are deeper beliefs and emotions focusing on guilt: a narrative which given the right person-centred approach may be revealed.

The ABC model can be extended now to include **'D'** Disputations of beliefs: this can be supported by the dialogue with healthcare professionals to challenge their *Beliefs* to create new *Consequences*, which then leads to adaption and implementation of **'E'** Effective new beliefs. In the scenario with the retained placenta, it would be useful for the clinician to provide professional challenge to her evaluation of being a failure by using supporting evidence from the notes, explaining the difference between an induction of labour and a spontaneous labour, the mechanism for a retained placenta, how the physical aspects of labour impacted on her physical fitness and the demands of feeding and caring for a newborn infant. As in Chapter 4, validation of her feelings is also important. As part of the dialogue, there needs to be an exploration of certain scenarios and how the woman and her partner might apply some coping mechanisms; for instance, if there is a repeat occurrence of a retained placenta and exploring how it might be experienced differently.

In a first birth, everything is a new experience: contractions, hospital care, bodily reactions, becoming a mother, breastfeeding, as well as learning new skills and knowledge. Women often need reminding just how physically and emotionally hard first-time childbirth and motherhood can be, but it will always be unique to a first birth. The anxiety of becoming a mother, the change in family dynamics, learning to understand what her baby needs, knowing what to do and when, most of this anxiety and learning is removed or reduced second time. As a result, even if a retained placenta occurs again, the mother and her partner will be dealing with it from a very different base: a potentially much stronger, more resilient base.

Anecdotally, clinicians are wary of setting women up to fail and not wanting to be blamed by women if, for instance, a repeat manual removal of placenta occurs or labour ends in an emergency CS. Additionally, as empathic clinicians, we can become sympathetic to a woman's previous story of birth trauma and feel a need to comply with a solution that appears to take away the anxiety and provide what we believe to be immediate relief to the woman by agreeing to a CS without understanding the fuller picture and perpetuating the woman's belief that she cannot cope with labour. A coping-orientated counselling style is about enabling women to tolerate uncertainty whilst increasing their self-confidence in dealing and coping with whatever occurs along the childbirth journey, rather than an assertion that everything is likely to go well this time. In a study which employed crisis-orientated counselling in a patient-centred approach (Nerum, 2006), 86 per cent of women changed their mind and decided on a vaginal birth. Women were then followed up at two–four years after birth. What is particularly interesting about this study is that even when labour ended in an emergency caesarean section, the women still expressed positive feelings about having managed their thinking and prepared for a vaginal birth. In the small group of women who continued with a planned CS, they commented that their psychological difficulties remained unresolved. In addition, having a CS for fear of birth does not guarantee a positive birth experience (Karlstrom et al, 2011).

Flexible plans

Whatever mode of birth women choose, a plan of care should be documented in the notes. This has been shown to reduce uncertainty in women who have had a previous traumatic experience and fosters a sense of control (Greenfield et al, 2019). Traditional birth plans, whereby all women are encouraged to plan for birth, have not always been used with the best intention (Whitford et al, 2014) and in areas where they are not valued or seen as part of routine care can be viewed negatively by staff (Grant et al, 2010). However, the types of plans we would advocate are not prescriptive. They are intended to help a busy clinician understand the reason for the fear or anxiety and what behaviours/actions would be helpful this time and what elements are important to a woman's psychological safety, for instance being kept fully informed and not being left alone without understanding why and for how long. Additionally, other factors such as environmental considerations and being free to adopt different positions are important to women. From experience, staff appreciate having this 'heads up' when women arrive in labour, with midwives valuing easily accessible information which highlights particular anxieties (Whitford et al, 2014). To make the plan more visible and to highlight anxiety issues on admission, a 'think pink' sticker on the notes to alert staff to mental health vulnerabilities has evaluated well (McKenzie-McHarg et al, 2014). Additionally, midwives need to feel confident in negotiating plans of care that may not follow local or national guidance, including the ability to support informed decision making, for instance negotiating place of birth. Interventions like this are aimed at keeping the internal locus of control with the woman and increase her feeling of competence and confidence. The obstetrician is also an important part in this process, especially if there are medical or obstetric risk factors. As a whole, the support should be collaborative and inclusive with the final decisions around mode of birth flexible throughout the journey.

Choice is not a stable entity; how a woman chooses to give birth will potentially change over the course of the pregnancy (Kingdon et al, 2009). When a woman who has had a previous vaginal birth asks for a CS at the midwifery booking assessment, how the midwife responds is crucial and we would suggest that unless there is a reason for needing to see an obstetrician, an obstetric consultation at this point should be avoided for the reasons stated earlier. The first intervention at this point is identification and immediate response by the community midwife, and this should include the following:

- Acknowledgement of the request and its importance to the woman
- Brief exploration of the reasons and validation of feelings
- Arrangement of a follow-up date to talk through the request or refer onwards depending on local service provision

It is important not to dismiss the request or try to talk the woman out of it. In maternity units that have a shared philosophy and understanding around childbirth fear and maternal request CS, the next part should ideally be a psychologically informed stepped care model with women having access to an appropriately trained midwife and, if needed, a psychologist. Working together with the woman, the psychologist and the midwife should have roles that complement each other to ensure that each part of any intervention is realistic, psychologically informed and deliverable.

Conclusion

How we support women with pregnancy-related anxiety and a fear of childbirth is complex and challenging. Interventions need to offer the woman a chance to reflect upon her situation, validate previous experience, reappraise and ultimately to feel supported. Using her own resources and other resources available, the result may be continued avoidance of the previous emotional turmoil including choosing a CS or she will become aware of, and process her experiences, with the possibility of choosing a vaginal birth (Nerum, 2006). How she chooses to give birth and our response to this are important; as clinicians we too have conscious and unconscious expectations and attitudes towards women and how they should give birth. Ultimately, the woman needs to feel supported, listened to and positive about approaching labour and birth.

References

Alio, A., Mbah, A., Grunsten, R. & Salihu, H. (2011). Teenage pregnancy and the influence of paternal involvement on fetal outcomes. *J Pediatr Adolesc Gynecol*, 24(6), 404–409.

Awad, O. & Bühling, K. (2011). Fathers in the delivery room: Results of a survey. *Geburtshilfe Frauenheilkd*, 71, 511–517.

Bandura, A. (1997). *Social learning theory*. Englewood Cliffs, NJ: Prentice Hall.

Bauer, A., Parsonage, M., Knapp, M., Lemmi, V. & Adelaja, B. (2014) The costs of perinatal mental health problems. *Centre for Mental Health and LSE.*

Bayrampour, H., Ali, E., McNeil, D. A., Benzies, K., MacQueen, G. & Tough, S. (2016). Pregnancy-related anxiety: A concept analysis. *Int J Nurs Stud*, 55, 115–130.

Beck, A. T. (1976). *Cognitive therapy and the emotional disorder survey*. Oxford: International Universities Press.

Birthrights (2018). Maternal request caesarean. Available online: https://birthrights.org.uk/wp-content/uploads/2018/08/Final-Birthrights-MRCS-Report-2108-1.pdf [Accessed 8 July 2019].

Brown, J. L., Sheffield, D., Leary, M. R. & Robinson, M. E. (2003). Social support and experimental pain. *Psychosomatic Medicine*, 65(2), 276–283.

Bryant, J., Porter, M., Tracy, S. K. & Sullivan, E. A. (2007). Caesarean birth: Consumption, safety, order, and good mothering. *Soc Sci Med*, 65(6), 1192–1201.

Caplan, G. (1964). *Principles of preventive psychiatry*. New York: Basic Books.

Carleton, R. N., Norton, M. A. & Asmundson, G. J. (2007). Fearing the unknown: A short version of the Intolerance of Uncertainty Scale. *J Anxiety Disord*, 21(1), 105–117.

Cherak, S. J., Giesbrecht, G. F., Metcalfe, A., Ronksley, P. E. & Malebranche, M. E. (2018). The effect of gestational period on the association between maternal prenatal salivary cortisol and birth weight: A systematic review and meta-analysis. *Psychoneuroendocrinology*, 94, 49–62.

Dehghani, M., Sharpe, L. & Khatibi, A. (2014). Catastrophizing mediates the relationship between fear of pain and preference for elective caesarean section. *European Journal of Pain*, 18(4), 582–589.

Dencker, A., Nilsson, C., Begley, C., Jangsten, E., Mollberg, M., Patel, H., Wigert, H., Hessman, E., Sjoblom, H. & Sparud-Lundin, C. (2019). Causes and outcomes in studies of fear of childbirth: A systematic review. *Women Birth*, 32(2), 99–111.

DiPietro, J. A., Ghera, M. M., Costigan, K. & Hawkins, M. (2009). Measuring the ups and downs of pregnancy stress. *Journal of Psychosomatic Obstetrics and Gynecology*, 25(3–4), 189–201.

Dugas, M. J., Hedayati, M., Karavidas, A., Buhr, K., Francis, K. & Phillips, N. A. (2005). Intolerance of uncertainty and information processing: Evidence of biased recall and interpretations. *Cognitive Therapy and Research*, 29(1), 57–70.

Dunkel Schetter, C. & Tanner, L. (2012). Anxiety, depression and stress in pregnancy: Implications for mothers, children, research, and practice. *Curr Opin Psychiatry*, 25(2), 141–148.

Dweik, D. & Sluijs, A. M. (2015). What is underneath the cesarean request? *Acta Obstet Gynecol Scand*, 94(11), 1153–1155.

Ellis, A. (1994) *Reason and emotion in psychotherapy*. Secaucus, NJ: Lyle Stuart.

Fenwick, J., Gamble, J. & Hauck, Y. (2006). Reframing birth: A consequence of cesarean section. *Journal of Advanced Nursing*, 56(2), 121–130.

Fenwick, J., Gamble, J., Nathan, E., Bayes, S. & Hauck, Y. (2009). Pre- and postpartum levels of childbirth fear and the relationship to birth outcomes in a cohort of Australian women. *Journal of Clinical Nursing*, 18(5), 667–677.

Fenwick, J., Staff, L., Gamble, J., Creedy, D. K. & Bayes, S. (2010) .Why do women request caesarean section in a normal, healthy first pregnancy? *Midwifery*, 26(4), 394–400.

Fenwick, J., Toohill, J., Gamble, J., Creedy, D. K., Buist, A., Turkstra, E., Sneddon, A., Scuffham, P. A. & Ryding, E. L. (2015). Effects of a midwife psycho-education intervention to reduce childbirth fear on women's birth outcomes and postpartum psychological wellbeing. *BMC Pregnancy Childbirth*, 15, 284.

Fisher, C., Hauck, Y. & Fenwick, J. (2006). How social context impacts on women's fears of childbirth: A Western Australian example. *Social Science and Medicine*, 63(1), 64–75.

Flink, I. K., Mroczek, M. Z., Sullivan, M. J. & Linton, S. J. (2009). Pain in childbirth and postpartum recovery: The role of catastrophizing. *Eur J Pain*, 13(3), 312–316.

Foa, E. B., Huppert, J. D. & Cahill, S. P. (2006). Emotional processing theory: An update. In B. O. Rothmaum (Ed.), *Pathological anxiety: Emotional processing in aetiology and treatment*. New York: Guildford Press, 3–24.

Garthus-Niegel, S., Knoph, C., Von Soest, T., Nielsen, C. S. & Eberhard-Gran, M. (2014) The role of labor pain and overall birth experience in the development of posttraumatic stress symptoms: A longitudinal cohort study. *Birth*, 41(1), 108–115.

Garthus-Niegel, S., Storksen, H. T., Torgersen, L., Von Soest, T. & Eberhard-Gran, M. (2011). The Wijma Delivery Expectancy/Experience Questionnaire – a factor analytic study. *Journal of Psychosomatic Obstetrics and Gynecology*, 32(3), 160–163.

Grant, R., Sueda, A. & Kaneshiro, B. (2010). Expert opinion vs. patient perception of obstetrical outcomes in labouring women with birth plans. *J Reprod Med*, 55, 31–35.

Green, J. M. & Baston, H. A. (2003). Feeling in control during labor: Concepts, correlates, and consequences. *Birth*, 30(4), 235–247.

Green, J. M. & Baston, H. A. (2007). Have women become more willing to accept obstetric interventions and does this relate to mode of birth? Data from a prospective study. *Birth*, 34, 6–13.

Greenfield, M., Jomeen, J. & Glover, L. (2019). "It can't be like last time" – choices made in early pregnancy by women who have previously experienced a traumatic birth. *Front Psychol*, 10, 56.

Haines, H., Pallant, J., Karlström, A. & Hildingsson, I. (2011). Cross-cultural comparison of levels of childbirth-related fear in an Australian and Swedish sample. *Midwifery*, 27(4), 560–567.

Halvorsen, L., Nerum, H., Sorlie, T. & Oian, P. (2010). Does counsellor's attitude influence change in a request for a caesarean in women with fear of birth? *Midwifery*, 26(1), 45–52.

Harpel, T. S. (2008). Fear of the unknown: Ultrasound and anxiety about fetal health. *Health (London)*, 12(3), 295–312.

Hildingsson, I., Karlstrom, A., Rubertsson, C. & Haines, H. (2019). Women with fear of childbirth might benefit from having a known midwife during labour. *Women Birth*, 32(1), 58–63.

Hildingsson, I., Rubertsson, C., Karlstrom, A. & Haines, H. (2018). Caseload midwifery for women with fear of birth is a feasible option. *Sex Reprod Healthc*, 16, 50–55.

Hodgkinson, E. L., Smith, D. M. & Wittkowski, A. (2014). Women's experiences of their pregnancy and postpartum body image: A systematic review and meta-synthesis. *BMC Pregnancy and Childbirth*, 14(1), 330.

Hofberg, K. & Ward, M. R. (2003). Fear of pregnancy and childbirth. *Postgraduate Medical Journal*, 79(935), 505–510.

Hornstein, E. A. & Eisenberger, N. I. (2017). Unpacking the buffering effect of social support figures: Social support attenuates fear acquisition. *PLoS One*, 12(5), e0175891.

Huizink, A. C., Menting, B., Oosterman, M., Verhage, M. L., Kunseler, F. C. & Schuengel, C. (2014). The interrelationship between pregnancy-specific anxiety and general anxiety across pregnancy: A longitudinal study. *J Psychosom Obstet Gynaecol*, 35(3), 92–100.

Jack, D. C. & Ali, A. (2010). *Silencing the self across cultures: Depression and gender in the social world.* Oxford: University Press.

Junge, C., von Soest, T., Weidner, K., Seidler, A., Eberhard-Gran, M. & Garthus-Niegel, S. (2018). Labor pain in women with and without severe fear of childbirth: A population-based, longitudinal study. *Birth*, 45(4), 469–477.

Karlstrom, A., Nystedt, A. & Hildingsson, I. (2011). A comparative study of the experience of childbirth between women who preferred and had a caesarean section and women who preferred and had a vaginal birth. *Sexual and Reproductive Healthcare*, 2(3), 93–99.

Kingdon, C., Neilson, J., Singleton, V., Gyte, G., Hart, A., Gabbay, M. & Lavender, T. (2009). Choice and birth method: Mixed-method study of caesarean delivery for maternal request. *BJOG*, 116(7), 886–895.

Kramer, M. S., Lydon, J., Seguin, L., Goulet, L., Kahn, S. R. & McNamara, H. (2009). Stress pathways to spontaneous preterm birth: The role of stressors, psychological distress, and stress hormones. *Am J Epidemiology*, 169(1319–1326).

Larsson, B., Karlstrom, A., Rubertsson, C. & Hildingsson, I. (2015). The effects of counseling on fear of childbirth. *Acta Obstet Gynecol Scand*, 94(6), 629–636.

Larsson, B., Karlstrom, A., Rubertsson, C. & Hildingsson, I. (2016). Counseling for childbirth fear-a national survey. *Sex Reprod Healthc*, 8, 82–87.

Littleton, H. L., Breitkopf, C. R. & Berenson, A. B. (2007). Correlates of anxiety symptoms during pregnancy and association with perinatal out-comes: A meta-analysis. *Am J. Obste. Gynecol*, 196(5), 424–432.

Longworth, M. K., Furber, C. & Kirk, S. (2015). A narrative review of fathers' involvement during labour and birth and their influence on decision making. *Midwifery*, 31(9), 844–857.

Lukasse, M., Schei, B., Ryding, E. L. & Bidens Study, G. (2014). Prevalence and associated factors of fear of childbirth in six European countries. *Sexual and Reproductive Healthcare*, 5(3), 99–106.

McKenzie-McHarg, K., Crockett, M., Olander, E. & Ayer, S. (2014). Think pink! A sticker alert system for psychological distress or vulnerability during pregnancy. *British Journal of Midwifery*, 22(8), 590–595.

McMahon, C. A., Boivin, J., Gibson, F. L., Hammarberg, K., Wynter, K. & Saunders, D. (2013). Pregnancy-specific anxiety ART conception and infant temperament at 4 months post-partum. *Human Reproduction*, 28, 997–1005.

Meyer, S. (2013). Control in childbirth: A concept analysis and synthesis. *Journal of Advanced Nursing*, 69(1), 218–228.

Nama, V. & Wilcock, F. (2011). Caesarean section on maternal request: Is justification necessary? *The Obstetrician and Gynaecologist*, 13, 263–269.

Nerum, H., Halvorsen, L., Sorlie, T. & Oian, P. (2006). Maternal request for cesarean section due to fear of birth: Can it be changed through crisis-oriented counseling? *Birth – Issues in Perinatal Care*, 33(3), 221–228.

Newham, J., Wittkowski, A., Hurley, J., Aplin J. D. & Westwood, M. (2014). Effects of antenatal yoga on maternal anxiety and depression: A randomized controlled trial. *Depression and Anxiety*, 31, 631–640.

NHS England (2019). *NHS Long Term Plan*. London: NHS England. Available online: www.longtermplan.nhs.uk/wp-content/uploads/2019/01/nhs-long-term-plan-june-2019.pdf [Accessed 17 June 2019].

NICE (2011). *Caesarean section (CG132)*. London: NICE.

NICE (2014). Antenatal and postnatal mental health: Clinical management and service guidance CG192. London: NICE.

Nilsson, C., Hessman, E., Sjoblom, H., Dencker, A., Jangsten, E., Mollberg, M., Patel, H., Sparud-Lundin, C., Wigert, H. & Begley, C. (2018). Definitions, measurements and prevalence of fear of childbirth: A systematic review. *BMC Pregnancy Childbirth*, 18(1), 28.

O'Connell, M. A., Leahy-Warren, P., Khashan, A. S., Kenny, L. C. & O'Neill, S. M. (2017). Worldwide prevalence of tocophobia in pregnant women: Systematic review and meta-analysis. *Acta Obstet Gynecol Scand*, 96(8), 907–920.

Oglesby, M. E., Boffa, J. W., Short, N. A., Raines, A. M. & Schmidt, N. B. (2016) Intolerance of uncertainty as a predictor of post-traumatic stress symptoms following a traumatic event. *J Anxiety Disord*, 41, 82–87.

Olieman, R. M., Siemonsma, F., Bartens, M. A., Garthus-Niegel, S., Scheele, F. & Honig, A. (2017). The effect of an elective cesarean section on maternal request on peripartum anxiety and depression in women with childbirth fear: A systematic review. *BMC Pregnancy Childbirth*, 17(1), 195.

Quartana, P. J., Campbell, C. M. & Edwards, R. R. (2009). Pain catastrophizing: A critical review. *Expert Rev Neurother*, 9(5), 745–758.

Rachman, S. (2001). Emotional processing, with special reference to post-traumatic stress disorder. *International Review of Psychiatry*, 13(3), 164–171.

Richens, Y., Hindley, C. & Lavender, T. (2015). A national online survey of UK maternity unit service provision for women with fear of birth. *British Journal of Midwifery*, 23(8), 574–579.

Richens, Y., Smith, D. M. & Lavender, D. T. (2018). Fear of birth in clinical practice: A structured review of current measurement tools. *Sex Reprod Healthc*, 16, 98–112.

Rollnick, S., Miller, W. R. & Butler, C. (2008). *Motivational interviewing in health care: Helping patients change behavior*. New York: Guildford Press.

Rondung, E., Ekdahl, J. & Sundin, O. (2018). Potential mechanisms in fear of birth: The role of pain catastrophizing and intolerance of uncertainty. *Birth*, 46(1), 61–68.

Rouhe, H., Salmela-Aro, K., Halmesmaki, E. & Saisto, T. (2009a). Fear of childbirth according to parity, gestational age and obstetric history. *BJOG – an International Journal of Obstetrics and Gynaecology*, 116(7), 1005–1006.

Rouhe, H., Salmela-Aro, K., Halmesmaki, E. & Saisto, T. (2009b). Fear of childbirth according to parity, gestational age, and obstetric history. *BJOG – an International Journal of Obstetrics and Gynaecology*, 116(1), 67–73.

Rustin, S. (2016). All British women have the right to a caesarean – they're not 'too posh to push', *Guardian*. Available online: www.theguardian.com/commentisfree/2016/mar/29/british-women-right-caesarean-too-posh-to-push [Accessed 8 July 2019].

Ryding, E. L., Lukasse, M., van Parys, A., Wangel, A., Karro, H., H., K., Schroll, A. & Schei, B. (2015). Fear of childbirth and risk of cesarean delivery: A cohort study in six European countries. *Birth*, 42(1), 48–55.

Saisto, T. & Halmesmaki, E. (2003). Fear of childbirth: A neglected dilemma. *Acta Obstetricia Et Gynecologica Scandinavica*, 82(3), 201–208.

Saisto, T., Ylikorkala, O. & Halmesmaki, E. (1999). Factors associated with fear of delivery in second pregnancies. *Obstetrics and Gynecology*, 94(5), 679–682.

Salmela-Aro, K., Read, S., Rouhe, H., Halmesmaki, E., Toivanen, R. M., Tokola, M. I. & Saisto, T. (2012). Promoting positive motherhood among nulliparous pregnant women with an intense fear of childbirth: RCT intervention. *Journal of Health Psychology*, 17(4), 520–534.

Sharpe, A. N., Waring, G. J., Rees, J., McGarry, K. & Hinshaw, K. (2015). Caesarean section at maternal request—the differing views of patients and healthcare professionals: A questionnaire based study. *Eur J Obstet Gynecol Reprod Biol*, 192, 54–60.

Sheen, K. & Slade, P. (2018). Examining the content and moderators of women's fears for giving birth: A meta-synthesis. *J Clin Nurs*, 27(13–14), 2523–2535.

Soderquist, J., Wijma, K. & Wijma, B. (2004). Traumatic stress in late pregnancy. *Journal of Anxiety Disorders*, 18(2), 127–142.

Staneva, A. A., Bogossian, F. & Wittkowski, A. (2015). The experience of psychological distress, depression, and anxiety during pregnancy: A meta-synthesis of qualitative research. *Midwifery*, 31(6), 563–573.

Staneva, A. A. & Wigginton, B. (2018). The happiness imperative: Exploring how women narrate depression and anxiety during pregnancy. *Feminism and Psychology*, 28(2), 173–193.

Stoll, K., Swift, E. M., Fairbrother, N., Nethery, E. & Janssen, P. (2018). A systematic review of nonpharmacological prenatal interventions for pregnancy-specific anxiety and fear of childbirth. *Birth*, 45(1), 7–18.

Storksen, H. T., Eberhard-Gran, M., Garthus-Niegel, S. & Eskild, A. (2012). Fear of childbirth; the relation to anxiety and depression. *Acta Obstetricia Et Gynecologica Scandinavica*, 91, 237–242.

Storksen, H. T., Garthus-Niegel, S., Vangen, S. & Eberhard-Gran, M. (2013). The impact of previous birth experiences on maternal fear of childbirth. *Acta Obstetricia Et Gynecologica Scandinavica*, 92(3), 318–324.

Striebich, S., Mattern, E. & Ayerle, G. M. (2018). Support for pregnant women identified with fear of childbirth (FOC)/tokophobia: A systematic review of approaches and interventions. *Midwifery*, 61, 97–115.

Ternstrom, E., Hildingsson, I., Haines, H. & Rubertsson, C. (2016). Pregnant women's thoughts when assessing fear of birth on the Fear of Birth Scale. *Women Birth*, 29(3), e44–49.

Toohill, J., Creedy, D. K., Gamble, J. & Fenwick, J. (2015). A cross-sectional study to determine utility of childbirth fear screening in maternity practice: An Australian perspective. *Women Birth*, 28(4), 310–316.

Toohill, J., Fenwick, J., Gamble, J., Creedy, D., Buist, A., Turkstra, E. & Ryding, E. (2014). A randomized controlled trial of a psycho-education intervention by midwives in reducing childbirth fear in pregnant women. *Birth*, 41(4), 384–394.

Turner, C. E., Young, J. M., Solomon, M. J., Ludlow, J., Benness, C. & Phipps, H. (2008). Vaginal delivery compared with elective caesarean section: The views of pregnant women and clinicians. *BJOG*, 115(12), 1494–502.

Uçar, T. & Golbasi, Z. (2018). Effect of an educational program based on cognitive behavioral techniques on fear of childbirth and the birth process. *Journal of Psychosomatic Obstetrics and Gynecology*, 40(2), 1–10.

Vallin, E., Nestander, H. & Wells, M. B. (2019). A literature review and meta-ethnography of fathers' psychological health and received social support during unpredictable complicated childbirths. *Midwifery*, 68, 48–55.

Van den Bergh, B. R., Mulder, E. J., Mennes, M. & Glover, V. (2005). Antenatal maternal anxiety and stress and the neurobehavioural development of the fetus and child: Links and possible mechanisms. A review. *Neurosci Biobehav Rev*, 29(2), 237–258.

Vlaeyen, J. & Linton, S. J. (2000). Fear-avoidance and its consequences in chronic musculoskeletal pain: A state of the art. *Pain*, 85, 317–332.

Waldenstrom, U., Hildingsson, I., Rubertsson, C. & Radestad, I. (2004). A negative birth experience: Prevalence and risk factors in a national sample. *Birth-Issues in Perinatal Care*, 31(1), 17–27.
Whitford, H., Entwistle, V. A., Teijingen, E., Aitchison, P. E., Davidson, T., Humphrey, T. & Tucker, J. (2014). Use of a birth plan within woman-held maternity records: A qualitative study with women and staff in Northeast Scotland. *Birth*, 41(3), 283–289.
Wijma, K. (2003). Why focus on 'fear of childbirth'? *Journal of Psychosomatic Obstetrics and Gynecology*, 24(3), 141–143.
Winton, E. C., Clark, D. M. & Edelmann, R. J. (1995). Social anxiety, fear of negative evaluation and the detection of negative emotion in others. *Behav Res Ther*, 33(2), 193–196.
Wulcan, A. C. & Nilsson, C. (2019). Midwives' counselling of women at specialised fear of childbirth clinics: A qualitative study. *Sex Reprod Healthc*, 19, 24–30.
Zar, M., Wijma, K. & Wijma, B. (2002). Relations between anxiety disorders and fear of childbirth during late pregnancy. *Clinical Psychology and Psychotherapy*, 9(2), 122–130.

7 Promoting staff resilience

Introduction

The National Maternity Review (NHS England, 2016) aims to increase personalised care, enable true choice and increase the provision of continuity of care and relational care which are linked to better outcomes for women and babies (Sandall et al, 2015). It is well known that respectful relationships and trust during labour are an important component of birth satisfaction (Waldenstrom et al, 2004) and feature in the post-partum narratives we hear. But none of us practise in a vacuum and being physically present is not enough: a compassionate clinician also needs to be mentally and emotionally present to address the needs of the patient (Leinweber & Rowe, 2010) and not as Berg et al (1996) describes 'absently present'. The essence of midwifery is being 'with woman', a reciprocal relationship based on trust but this requires midwives to feel valued, cared for and respected (Ball et al, 2002). In essence how we care is affected by our working environment and this is true across all healthcare organisations; the more positive the experiences of staff within the NHS, the better the outcomes are for the hospital and patients (West & Dawson, 2012). Women's narratives afford us an opportunity to reflect on our care practices through a difference lens, to gain greater understanding and to reflect, learn and adapt. This is crucial to maintaining and improving compassionate care, but if we are to get the experiences right for women in the longer term we need to understand and support staff in maintaining empathic, woman-centred care. An appreciation then of the current climate and culture in which we practice is necessary, including the discourse of risk and clinical governance and its effect on clinical decision making and practice.

Understanding how culture frames practice

Culture can be defined simply as 'the way things are done around here' (Kotter & Heskett, 2008) and with the majority of women giving birth in a hospital, how a midwife practises will be influenced by the leadership and ethos within the maternity unit and the relationship with the multi-disciplinary team. The consequence of dysfunctional relationships in maternity and its impact on safety is well documented (Kirkup, 2015). In addition, an environment that is hierarchal and not open to change can make it difficult for midwives to present choices and advocate for women (Hauck et al, 2016). Studies exploring the experiences of newly qualified midwives have repeatedly shown that new midwives feel an expectation to conform to the cultural identity of a unit even if that means compromising woman-centred care (Hobbs, 2012). Even midwives who have been qualified for a number of years have been found to take a passive role and conform to the norms of an institutionalised hospital culture (Sidebotham et al, 2015)

This is an important consideration as we know that choice and control during childbirth are important to women, and when present are linked to a positive evaluation of birth (Cook & Loomis, 2012; Hodnett, 2002). The element of control for each woman is subjective and variable. Green and Baston (2003) make two distinctions: *internal* control is the control a woman has over her body and *external* control the control she has over medical staff and decisions made in relation to her labour. Like the NHS Maternity review (NHS England, 2016), previous national policy (DH, 1993; 2007) has also respected the ideals of placing women at the heart of what we do, respecting wishes and choices around care provision and promoting a narrative that allows women to make choices outside of the recommended guidance, albeit through balanced and objective discussion. The midwife plays a pivotal role in communicating choice in labour and women expect and want midwives to act as their advocate in labour (Hallam et al, 2016).

Yet if midwives work within a system that does not embrace collaborative working and the ideals of women-centred care, then advocating for women can feel challenging and midwives may instead choose to practise 'with institution' rather than 'with woman' (Hunter, 2005). Or they choose when to advocate depending on who is on duty (Hauck et al, 2016). In this way, women's choices and wishes are marginalised to avoid professional conflict and challenge (Bedwell et al, 2015) and to align care instead with the expected cultural norms. There is also a sense of divided loyalties amongst midwives between the medical model and the midwifery model of supporting normal physiology, with midwives tending to adapt their own practice to conform with the culture of the maternity unit (O'Connell & Downe, 2009). Dynamic tensions between professional groups have also been shown in studies looking at intrapartum transfer from home or midwife-led units to an obstetric hospital (Ball et al, 2016; Kuliukas et al, 2017) and whilst the ethos of midwifery is to empower women and promote the normal physiology of labour it is often midwives themselves who perpetuate the discourse of the biomedical model and strict adherence to policy (Healy et al, 2016). For midwives who want to advocate for women there can then be a sense of disillusionment and frustration, often accompanied by workplace conflict and stress (Hunter, 2004). It can also leave midwives feeling a sense of guilt and betrayal, especially if they feel they have been complicit in disrespectful care (Leinweber et al, 2017a).

As well as the professional power dynamics, hospital governance structures have introduced the concept of risk management strategies to improve safety in healthcare. Today risk assessments are embedded throughout the maternity care pathway and risk reporting details every part of our everyday life in practice, from shoulder dystocia to needlestick injury. The term clinical negligence seems to be etched into our arteries. In a survey by the British Medical Association (BMA, 2018), 55 per cent of doctors stated that they worry about being unfairly blamed for errors and as a result 49 per cent reported that they practise defensively. In obstetric practice doctors have cited a fear of litigation as one of the main reasons for the rising caesarean section rates (Savage & Francome, 2007). The impact can be seen in the Birthplace in England study (Brocklehurst et al, 2011), which compared outcomes for 'low risk' women starting labour in four different environments: home, midwife led unit-alongside, midwife led unit-freestanding and obstetric unit. Using a composite primary outcome of perinatal mortality and intrapartum-related neonatal morbidities there were no significant differences in the odds of the primary outcome across all four birth setting (analysis by parity did show a higher incidence of the primary outcome in primiparous women planning birth at home). What is interesting about this study is the differing rates of intervention, with the chance of achieving a normal birth (birth without induction of labour, epidural or spinal anaesthesia, general anaesthesia, forceps or ventouse, caesarean section, or episiotomy) varying significantly from 58 per cent for planned obstetric unit births, 78 per cent in an alongside midwife-led unit and 88 per cent for planned home births.

In midwifery the perceived threat of litigation and complaints has been further linked to an erosion of midwives autonomy and inability to make decisions in labour, with midwives preferring instead to defer to an obstetrician (Everly, 2012; Healy et al, 2017). This has also led to midwives carrying out interventions in labour even if they disagree with the necessity (Seibold et al, 2010). When exploring defensive practice amongst midwives Symon (2000) found that the use of continuous electronic fetal monitoring (CEFM) when not medically indicated was commonly cited by midwives. The evidence base around CEFM without medical indication and the link to an increase in caesarean section and operative births without any differences in cerebral palsy, infant mortality or other standard measures of neonatal wellbeing has become more well known since this time with publication of the first Cochrane systematic review (Thacker et al, 2001) and has been echoed in all subsequent reviews (Alfirevic et al, 2017) and in national guidance (NICE, 2014) so it is worrying that in Healy's et al (2016) study midwives reported that even when not clinically indicated using CEFM would receive no institutional criticism whereas underutilisation would lead to recrimination if an adverse event occurred. This overuse of CEFM has been well documented as a fear response amongst midwives to ensure they have a defence just in case a complaint or claim ensues (Robertson & Thomson, 2016). In addition if women choose not to have CEFM when considered clinically relevant and as detailed in the maternity unit guidelines midwives will exercise a degree of professional persuasion and rather than advocating for women will ensure the responsibility for the decision is articulated and documented as resting solely with the woman (Robertson & Thomson, 2016). In a study exploring midwives fears, missing something that causes harm was ranked second highest, other factors included 'being watched and criticised' and litigation (Dahlen & Caplice, 2014). So whilst midwives may verbalise intention to practise in a collaborative model with women in reality there can be a professional tension resulting in midwives feeling unable to enact this in practice (O'Connell & Downe, 2009)

This is evident when trying to triangulate some of the narratives we hear from women with the midwives providing care often defending their position by saying 'but that's what the guideline says'. Of course it depends on the clinical scenario, but often we don't ask the right questions. From experience, when a woman chooses something outside of normal practice it is usually because she wants to avoid something else; sometimes when we endeavour to understand this part of the request it becomes easier to facilitate what she needs. From experience, this is frequently highlighted when women with co-morbidities ask to be cared for on the midwife led unit (MLU) in labour. When asked, 'tell me what it is that is important to you for your labour' rather than merely highlighting to her why she doesn't fit the criteria for 'low risk' MLU care, then these women will often reply using phrases such as needing a relaxed environment, needing to feel calm, being able to move freely and wanting to feel safe. All of this can and should be facilitated in any environment, and often that surprises women. Of course women often want to be on a MLU so they can use the pool and this is when as midwives, we need to be able to articulate what the evidence does and doesn't tell us, alongside the risk and benefits of being in water. This is challenging as often the required care is debatable within a 'grey area' and without clear evidence (Rowe, 2010). Sometimes women will modify their choices and, if not, midwives have a professional obligation to be that woman's advocate (NMC, 2009). Whilst hospital guidelines utilise best evidence, they are intended to guide practice, yet they are often interpreted by midwives as documents that must be adhered to for professional safety (Porter et al, 2007; Robertson & Thomson,

2016). This is in direct contrast to the definition of evidence-based medicine as originally introduced by Sackett (1997) which requires a triangulation of best external evidence, clinical expertise and patient values and preferences. This is why when we start to look at what affects a woman's experience of her labour and birth and on how we can improve care, we find that it is a multi-layered task.

None of these themes are new and formed part of the analysis done by (Ball et al, 2002) on why midwives leave the profession. All that is perhaps different today is our awareness of the problem and the resultant emotional toll on staff wellbeing. The WHELM study (Hunter et al, 2018) reported that midwives in the UK were suffering from high levels of stress, burnout and depression with two thirds of respondents stating that they had considered leaving the profession in the last six months. The emotionally demanding work of caring has been highlighted over the last decade by a growing number of studies looking at burn out and stress in healthcare workers (Adriaenssens et al, 2015; Ruotsalainen et al, 2015).

Stress, burnout and secondary traumatic stress

The terms *burnout* and *stress* tend to be used interchangeably and often wrapped around the concept of *compassion fatigue* with much debate as to whether they exist as separate entities or are interrelated, with one causing the other (Sinclair et al, 2017).

Burnout is one of the earliest used terms to describe workplace-related stress in the caring professions (Jackson & Maslach, 1982). It consists of emotional exhaustion, depersonalisation and negative thinking towards others (Pezaro et al, 2016; Yoshida & Sandall, 2013). Pezaro et al (2016) offers the simple explanation that as the emotional stores of the midwife run low so burnout can ensue along with the ability to care compassionately.

The concept of *compassion fatigue* is attributed to Figley (1995), who wanted to develop a model that could predict the onset of compassion fatigue in psychotherapists. Figley (1995) proposed that part of the therapist's empathic response to the clients suffering involves projecting themselves into the client's perspective. The emotional energy that this requires causes compassion stress which if not contained or recognised can lead to compassion fatigue. There is some criticism that this is very linear and somewhat fatalistic view of empathic caring as it implies that compassion fatigue is almost an inevitable component of providing empathic care, furthermore its widespread adoption to nursing and midwifery has been questioned (Sinclair et al, 2017). More recently, compassion fatigue in midwives has been linked to what has been coined a 'moral distress' (Ledoux, 2015) to describe workplace stressors occurring when staff are unable to give the care they value and believe is necessary. This in turn can cause feelings of guilt and concern for the quality of care afforded to a client (Ledoux, 2015). In a meta-synthesis exploring the evidence around compassion fatigue in nursing Nolte et al (2017) found that compassion-fatigued nurses tended to distance themselves from others including any emotional attachment to patients as a way of coping.

Alongside workplace-related stress there is a growing body of evidence exploring post-traumatic stress (PTS) in healthcare professionals. In terms of prevalence, figures vary depending on methodology and measures, but the estimates nonetheless seem high. In the first UK-based survey exploring midwives experience of traumatic events 33 per cent of midwives had symptoms of post-traumatic stress disorder (PTSD), this was accompanied by emotional exhaustion and disengagement from women in their care (Sheen et al, 2015). In a survey of Australian midwives (Leinweber et al, 2017b) using a different measure, prevalence rates for PTSD were found to be 17 per cent.

This type of work-place related trauma is termed *secondary traumatic stress* and was also described originally by Figley (1995) before being replaced with the term *compassion fatigue* as Figley felt this was less derogatory (Beck, 2011). In the literature, the two terms are often used as separate entities or interchangeably. In essence, what is being described is a stress response to the act of providing an empathic connection with someone *who is* or *who has* endured trauma (Beck, 2011; Sinclair et al, 2017) and it can also occur from listening to traumatic events, for instance women's post-partum narratives of a traumatic birth (Sheen et al, 2015). In more recent times, compassion fatigue has been used to describe an emotional state which can evolve over time, whereas secondary trauma can result from being exposed to a single traumatic event (Leinweber & Rowe, 2010). However, like primary trauma it does not follow that exposure to a 'traumatic event' will result in symptoms of PTS or in compassion fatigue in all clinicians (Leinweber & Rowe, 2010). In a large meta-analysis of work-related critical incidents, de Boer et al (2011) found that hospital staff working in areas where incidents and emergencies happened frequently had a lower prevalence rate of trauma symptoms compared to staff in areas where emergencies were witnessed infrequently, with an assumption that where staff are drilled and trained to respond they may cope better in such circumstances.

The term *vicarious trauma* often used synonymously with *secondary trauma* has a slightly different meaning and relates to the actual effects of secondary trauma exposure on the clinician, described as a change to a person's world view, with feelings of low self-esteem, lack of trust in self and others, withdrawal and avoidance of others (Măirean & Turliuc, 2013).

For clinicians working in maternity, maternal morbidity and severe asphyxia of the newborn are the most frequently witnessed traumatic events (Wahlberg et al, 2017). In a Danish study (Schroder et al, 2016) with a good response rate from both obstetricians and midwives, 85 per cent of staff stated that they had been involved in a traumatic birth, defined as an event in which the infant or the mother suffered presumed permanent, severe and possibly fatal injuries related to the birth. But a *traumatic* event is not only defined as involvement in an adverse outcome or an emergency clinical scenario; yes, these scenarios often involve a heightened sense of anxiety, but they can also be rationalised cognitively over time as events that occur randomly. This is perhaps reflected in Schroder et al's (2016) findings that 65 per cent of respondents felt the critical incident made them a better midwife or doctor. This type of clinical adverse outcome is in direct contrast to perceived interpersonal trauma. As human beings working in a caring profession, our view of the world and what is right is thrown off-centre when we witness what we perceive to be a lack of compassion, whether directed to ourselves or to others: when this occurs it cognitively challenges our assumptions of safety and predictability of the world (Forbes et al, 2012). These types of interpersonal care-giving behaviours feature highly in studies examining trauma experiences of midwives, in particular witnessing disrespectful or abusive care (Leinweber et al, 2017a; Leinweber & Rowe, 2010; Rice & Warland, 2013), in Leinweber et al's (2017b) study, midwives witnessing this type of trauma had more PTS symptoms. Understanding why interpersonal trauma has a greater affect is very similar to the evidence discussed in Chapter 2 around how women can often make sense of random emergency events that occur in labour (as long as they are well handled and the woman feels safe) whilst struggle to makes sense of perceived unkindness by a healthcare professional who they trust implicitly to provide compassionate, safe care.

Whilst there is still some debate around definitions and how stress, burnout, PTS and compassion fatigue inter-relate, in essence they are all describing a psychological stress experienced by clinicians which may cause stress-type symptoms and an inability to maintain an empathic bond. In the majority of post-partum narratives we hear, a lack of effective communication features highly as does a perceived lack of compassion. When this happens women describe feeling a sense of helplessness, fear and abandonment which are often described in the evidence as contributing to PTSD post-birth (Beck, 2004).

This then highlights why it is important to understand the phenomena within the maternity setting and the possible implications for providing woman centred care if midwives feel unable to engage in a therapeutic relationship. The very nature of the role of the midwife is to provide a compassionate and empathic connection (Hunter et al, 2008) with mutual trust and respect. This is hugely important to women in how they view their pregnancy, birth and adaptation to motherhood (Dahlberg & Aune, 2013; Hodnett, 2002; Waldenstrom et al, 2004), yet it is also a key component in the development of secondary traumatic stress in staff (Beck, 2011). In essence if midwives feel unable to provide an empathic relationship this will have an impact on how women view and remember their care.

Understanding resilience

With stress being a major contributor of staff absence and staff retention rates falling in the NHS (NHS England, 2019), there is much interest in developing tools that support staff in dealing with stress and to foster emotional wellbeing (Health Education England, 2019). In a Cochrane systematic review (Ruotsalainen et al, 2015) looking at occupational stress in healthcare workers, fifty-eight studies were identified and fifty-four were randomised controlled trials. It identified low quality evidence that cognitive behavioural therapy (CBT) and mental and physical relaxation reduce stress and low quality evidence that changing work schedules may lead to a reduction in stress. Overall it concluded that more high quality studies are needed. Treating the symptoms is one element, but if the NHS is to make significant strides it needs to challenge the causes of workplace stress (West & Willis, 2015).

Following NHS organisational failings (Francis, 2013; Kirkup, 2015), the role of leadership within the NHS and its pivotal role in organisational culture has been much criticised. In response to this, The Kings Fund suggests that more collective leadership models are needed, aimed at giving frontline staff the autonomy and control to provide safe care (West et al, 2017). This high level of attention to culture, leadership and seeking to understand what keeps staff emotionally healthy is inter-related with the growing awareness that we need to foster and support the workforce to build resilience with the expectation that it will reduce the occurrence of stress and burnout.

The origins of our knowledge about resilience lies within the discipline of psychology and has become a common theme within midwifery and nursing texts (Cleary et al, 2018; Delgado et al, 2017; Hunter & Warren, 2014; Manomenidis et al, 2019). There are theoretically differing definitions of resilience, debated as being either a personality trait that helps individuals cope with adversity, a behavioural outcome occurring after trauma exposure that helps individuals to recover or a dynamic process in which an individual adapts and recovers rapidly following trauma (Hu et al, 2015)

One of the problems with identifying resilience solely as a personality trait is that there is often a value judgement placed on individuals who are perceived as lacking in resilience versus those that 'have what it takes' (Luthar et al, 2000). It also assumes that someone who is labelled as resilient will always cope with adversity – that it is a fixed entity – and this is not true. In terms of exploring how resilience can be promoted and supported within midwifery, we prefer the construct of resilience as a dynamic developmental process (Achenbach, 1993). Seen in this way as a cognitive process there is some overlap with the evidence around post-traumatic growth (discussed in Chapter 2) and used in this context asserts that staff can benefit from a positive cognitive adjustment following an incident or experience if the conditions are right. Resilience describes a resistance in the face of adversity (Smith, 1999), yet evidence suggests that whilst the features of resilience are recognised as being able to draw upon effective resources at the time to protect the self from harm, there is also the ability to recover from harm (Luthar et al, 2000), as resilience is malleable over time as one adapts after experiencing stressful events (Meredith et al, 2011). We often share with staff the metaphor of resilience being like a plumb line: events and experiences may knock us 'off-centre' but resilience is our ability to return to our centre. Studies have shown that high levels of resilience measured in individuals are associated with lower levels of stress, anxiety and depression (Hu et al, 2015; Mautner et al, 2013) and PTSD (Thompson et al, 2018). Understanding then how resilience can be strengthened and what factors are protective would seem essential to ensuring a continued empathic connection with women and in retaining staff.

Building resilience in the workforce

Environmental

The space in which care is provided is important. Within the midwives usual intrapartum repository is the skill of creating an ambient and calm birth space to promote the physiological process of labour and release of oxytocin. As well as being crucial for maintaining adequate contractions in labour, oxytocin also plays a dynamic role within human behaviour, improving social interactions and emotional aspects of behaviour and so facilitating positive human relationships (Ishak et al, 2011). This benefits not only the woman but can also affect the midwives physiology, promoting a feeling of relaxation and sense of calmness (Hammond et al, 2013). Additionally high levels of resilience and compassionate care are associated with professional autonomy and a workplace that allows midwives to work to the ideals of 'with woman' rather than conforming to the demands of a busy obstetric led unit (Davis & Homer, 2016; McDonald et al, 2016). In Davis and Homer's (2016) study of midwives practising across a variety of settings in the UK and Australia the obstetric environment was described as 'busy work', whereby the midwives working on the labour ward were expected to do other work alongside providing one-to-one care in labour, appearing to be 'busy' was given high precedence. Whereas in home and birth centre settings midwives were able to behave in ways that were considered 'unprofessional' in the hospital, for instance taking off shoes and having a cup of tea with the family. Getting the ambience right for women to birth can also reduce workplace-related stress in midwives and enhance wellbeing at work (Davis & Homer, 2016; Hammond et al, 2017).

Influencing the organisational culture and the way models of care are delivered takes time. Midwives working in hospitals and the community require supportive measures to allow for safe ventilation of feelings. This must involve all maternity care workers, qualified staff and unqualified staff, and all areas of practice. Intrapartum care can be unpredictable and stressful yet so too can community working. All grades of staff working in all areas require the tools to maintain empathic relationships with women and to be able to enhance and maintain their own emotional health and wellbeing.

Self-compassion

In midwifery, Hunter and Warren (2014) provided the first study exploring how resilience is experienced in practice. The study describes midwives experiences of 'protective self-management' including the ability to recognise stress triggers as a key component of resilience building. In the study, this protective factor is linked to peer support, the ability to reflect and having a balanced, realistic view of expectations and limitations. This relates well to the concept of self-compassion which, when present, is linked to reduced cortisol levels and an ability to self-soothe (Rockliff et al, 2008). In Chapter 2 we discussed activation of the 'threat system' and this is also applicable to healthcare professionals. Working in areas that can be unpredictable and fast paced requires an individual to be able to self-soothe and potentially deactivate the 'threat response' (Beaumont et al, 2016).

Self-compassion is seen as an integral part of building resilience and maintaining compassion in practice. People who score highly on self-compassion are able to accept themselves for all inadequacies and failings and rather than disconnect from their suffering, accept it and seek to alleviate with self-kindness (Neff, 2003). Self-compassionate people are less likely to ruminate on negative thoughts and emotions and have a greater ability to cope with negative emotions (Heffernan et al, 2010). Thus greater self-compassion is associated with lower levels of anxiety and depression (Macbeth & Gumley, 2012) and lower levels of compassion fatigue and personal distress (Duarte et al, 2016). The evidence also suggests that self-compassion can be protective against PTSD (Beaumont et al, 2012) and reduces the incidence of burn out and compassion fatigue in healthcare staff (Dev et al, 2018). This is thought to be due to the way in which individuals are able to manage their own stress (Vigna et al, 2018).

Describing self-compassion, Neff (2003) describes three interacting components, each with a negative and positive pole. (See Box 7.1.)

BOX 7.1 Interacting components of self-compassion (Neff, 2003)

Self-kindness versus Self-judgement	Rather than criticising and judging oneself, practice unconditional acceptance and understanding
Common humanity versus Isolation	All people fail and/or make mistakes Accept that imperfection is a way of life
Mindfulness versus Over-identification	Be conscientiously aware of painful experiences. Don't ignore or exaggerate painful thoughts and emotions

Self-compassion is also interlinked with mindfulness-based interventions (Kuyken et al, 2010) and is seen to be a robust resilience factor when feelings of personal inadequacy invade the psyche (Macbeth & Gumley, 2012). In addition being self-compassionate does not mean that you simply accept a lower standard of self, or become complacent, in fact studies suggest that it improves self-improvement motivation, motivating people to improve after personal failure and not being afraid to try again (Breines & Chen, 2012).

Restorative supervision

Clinical Supervision is widely embedded within counselling and psychology services and in clinical areas known for being emotionally stressful, such as palliative care and mental health (Butterworth et al, 1998). This is not to be confused with safeguarding supervision, which has been embedded in health visiting and midwifery as part of child protection. More recently with the increasing awareness around stress and burnout in midwifery, group clinical supervision sessions have been evaluated positively by midwives (Love et al, 2017). The authors note, however, that the term clinical supervision implies assessment of practice when in fact the sessions are aimed towards encouraging reflection and support. In the UK, clinical supervision is receiving increased attention through the new model of A-EQUIP by NHS England (2017), which has been developed after statutory supervision of midwives ended in March 2017. The A-EQUIP model (an acronym for Advocating and Educating for Quality Improvement) aims to 'build personal and professional resilience of midwives, enhance quality of care and support preparedness for appraisal and professional revalidation' (NHS England, 2017). The A-EQUIP model utilises a supervision model based on Proctors work (1986), which includes the following: *formative* (increase knowledge and skills), *normative* (monitoring quality and professional practice) and *restorative* (to enhance health and wellbeing). The final arm of the model is *personal action for quality improvement.* To deliver this model NHS England has developed the Professional Midwifery Advocate (PMA) role. In Proctor's model (1986), the *normative* and *formative* elements tend to focus on increasing knowledge, clinical competency and performance. The part of the model which we feel warrants particular attention is the evidence around the *restorative* arm of clinical supervision, especially when considering the emotional work of midwifery (Hunter, 2005).

The *restorative* function of supervision has the addition of psychological support including listening, supporting and challenging the supervisee to improve their own capacity to cope (Proctor 1986), which resonates somewhat with the elements discussed in Chapter 3 and the humanistic principles of active listening. If it is done well, restorative clinical supervision (RCS) offers a safe space to reflect on care and process the emotional demands of the role and has been shown to reduce stress and burnout in a maternity workforce (Wallbank, 2013). RCS also aims to increase personal confidence and self-efficacy and address stress management techniques, all of which are considered important elements for enhancing resilience in midwifery; as Hunter and Warren (2014) assert resilience is not just about survival, it is about learning and finding healthy ways to cope. Seen in this way, resilience can be developed and practised.

In Chapter 6 we discussed using the ABC model (Ellis, 1994) and this can be used in supervision sessions or for individual staff members to use within reflections. The model can help individuals to understand personal responses to stress and adversity in the workplace. As discussed previously it is our emotional response to an event that drives the subsequent behavioural action. Sessions can be on a one-to-one basis or in a group. A recent systematic review looking at interventions to improve resilience among health professionals has shown that resilience awareness workshops delivered in groups is an effective intervention (Cleary et al, 2018). One of the benefits of delivering RCS to a small group is that it enables staff to share experiences with colleagues and/or discuss difficult scenarios, with the prevalence of twelve-hour shifts the overlapping of staff shifts has gone and anecdotally the opportunity to share and debrief seems to be lost. In a group scenario, staff will be aware that they are not alone and there can be a sense of relief to hear that others in the group are experiencing the same challenges and/or self-doubt, hence normalising feelings and emotions (Sheppard et al, 2018). This is especially important with staff members who have a propensity towards self-criticism which is linked to psychological morbidity, including depression and anxiety disorders (Beaumont et al, 2012). Self-critical individuals tend to feel unworthy and inferior to peers (Neff, 2003), fearing disapproval from others and a loss of acceptance (Blatt & Zuroff, 1992).

CASE STUDY 7.1 Charlotte: a newly qualified midwife

Whilst still in her preceptorship period, Charlotte was working a night shift on labour ward, she had been enjoying all her shifts so far and was working with a really good supportive team. Later in the night she was asked to move to the antenatal ward for the rest of her night shift. She had not yet worked on the antenatal ward as a qualified member of staff but she liked the co-ordinator who asked her and whilst she felt scared, she agreed to the move. The ward was busy and after only a very quick handover Charlotte answered the call bell to a young woman who had been admitted earlier in day with threatened pre-term labour at less than thirty weeks. The woman appeared comfortable but gave a good history of her contractions becoming painful again so Charlotte decided to start a CTG (fetal heart rate monitor) to assess what was happening. Leaving the room to find a CTG she was distracted by another woman whose labour was being induced and who was asking for pain relief. It was some time before she returned with a CTG. When she arrived back the woman was visibly uncomfortable and said she wanted to push. Pulling back the covers Charlotte could see that her waters had broken and birth was imminent. Charlotte immediately pulled the emergency buzzer and the first midwife who arrived at the scene asked her if she had called the neonatal team. Charlotte replied no and as more staff members arrived started to feel more out of her depth, she was asked how many weeks (gestation) and if it was definitely cephalic (head down) Charlotte didn't have the information to hand, she felt overwhelmed and she was aware of her heart beat 'like it was ringing in my ears … I felt physically sick'. Her previous self-confidence during her time on labour ward had left her and she felt totally inadequate 'I felt like a fraud; I should have known what to do …' The senior midwife on duty appeared calm and took charge with authority. There was a good outcome, the baby delivered very quickly and was taken by the neonatal team to the special care unit. Charlotte was able to stay with the woman afterwards and help her to emotionally process what had happened, call her partner, shower and then spend time with her baby on the special care unit.

This was her last night shift and she wasn't due back at work for five days. During that time she slept badly and kept returning to the scenario. She judged herself against that senior midwife who was so calm and in control, she perceived her actions that night as inadequate and admitted that it 'knocked all my self-confidence out the window'. When she arrived back on a day shift, she saw the senior midwife from that night, who immediately started a conversation about their last night shift and apologised for not being able to talk to her at the end of the shift. She praised Charlotte for her actions and said, 'that was a tough scenario for any midwife let alone someone still in her preceptorship period'. The senior midwife encouraged Charlotte to re-evaluate her own self-criticisms and to view her performance against the expected actions of a newly qualified midwife. When the senior midwife admitted 'you know I was panicked too … it doesn't matter how long you have been qualified … untoward events like that are scary … as you get older you develop a mask that gives you a perceived air of confidence … but underneath … yes it is scary … and that's normal … otherwise we wouldn't respond'. This was hugely healing for Charlotte.

Charlotte's narrative (Case Study 7.1) highlights the importance of connectedness, as humans we desire connection with others throughout the life span, developing and sustaining healthy relationships that foster growth and a sense of safety and wellbeing which can in itself be a healing mechanism (Jordan, 2010). It also resonates with the ever enlightening work of Brene Brown (2006) around women and shame resilience theory: '… one of the most important benefits of developing empathy and connection with others is recognizing how the experiences that make us feel the most alone, and even isolated, are often the most universal experiences' (p. 49).

In addition to shared experiences and meeting the *restorative* function of clinical supervision, a group supervision model facilitated by an appropriately trained PMA can also fulfil the additional functions of *formative* and *normative* clinical supervision by allowing participants to self-reflect and reframe issues (formative), to discuss and critique practice and improve care (normative). If it is done well, a group RCS session helps individuals to feel accepted amongst their peers despite their own perceived inner failings and experiencing, too, a sense of shared experience and support (Sheppard et al, 2018). In Love et al's (2017) study exploring clinical supervision for midwives, they draw parallels between the supportive and developmental focus of what they term 'reflective clinical supervision' and the wellness framework and philosophy of midwifery care.

Conclusion

Whilst there is much attention in the NHS around building a compassionate workforce and improving resilience, there are many facets within the concept of resilience that potentially make interventions challenging and it is unlikely there will be a one-size-fits-all model. There is certainly more evidence needed to understand interventions that work for the NHS (Cleary et al, 2018). Supporting staff in finding and learning healthy ways to cope and thrive rather than merely surviving (Wendt et al, 2011) is one aspect. In addition, as maternity services seek to improve continuity and relational care, it is vital that we also reflect on the environment and culture in which care is provided to ensure that they too are conducive to maintaining and encouraging humanistic, empathic relationships with women.

References

Achenbach, T. M. (1993). Taxonomy and comorbidity of conduct problems: Evidence from empirically based approaches. *Dev Psychopathol*, 5(1–2), 51–64.

Adriaenssens, J., De Gucht, V. & Maes, S. (2015). Determinants and prevalence of burnout in emergency nurses: A systematic review of 25 years of research. *International Journal of Nursing Studies*, 52(2), 649–661.

Alfirevic, Z., Gyte, G. M. L., Cuthbert, A. & Devane, D. (2017). Continuous cardiotocography (CTG) as a form of electronic fetal monitoring (EFM) for fetal assessment during labour. *Cochrane Database of Systematic Reviews* (2).

Ball, C., Hauck, Y., Kuliukas, L., Lewis, L. & Doherty, D. (2016). Under scrutiny: Midwives' experience of intrapartum transfer from home to hospital within the context of a planned homebirth in Western Australia. *Sexual and Reproductive Healthcare*, 8, 88–93.

Ball, L., Curtis, P. & Kirkham, M. (2002). *Why do midwives leave?* London: The Royal College of Midwives.

Beaumont, E., Durkin, M., Hollins Martin, C. J. & Carson, J. (2016). Compassion for others, self-compassion, quality of life and mental well-being measures and their association with compassion fatigue and burnout in student midwives: A quantitative survey. *Midwifery*, 34, 239–244.

Beaumont, E., Galpin, A. & Jenkins, P. (2012). 'Being kinder to myself': A prospective comparative study, exploring post-trauma therapy outcome measures, for two groups of clients, receiving either cognitive behaviour therapy or cognitive behaviour therapy and compassionate mind training. *Counselling Psychol Rev*, 27(1), 31–43.

Beck, C. T. (2004). Post-traumatic stress disorder due to childbirth: The aftermath. *Nursing Research*, 53(4), 216–224.

Beck, C. T. (2011). Secondary traumatic stress in nurses: A systematic review. *Arch Psychiatr Nurs*, 25(1), 1–10.

Bedwell, C., McGowan, L. & Lavender, T. (2015). Factors affecting midwives' confidence in intrapartum care: A phenomenological study. *Midwifery*, 31(1), 170–176.

Berg, M., Lundgren, I., Hermansson, E. & Wahlberg, V. (1996). Women's experience of the encounter with the midwife during childbirth. *Midwifery*, 12(1), 11–15.

Blatt, S. J. & Zuroff, D. C. (1992). Interpersonal relatedness and self-definition: Two prototypes for depression. *Clinical Psychology Review*, 12(5), 527–562.

BMA (2018). *Caring, supportive, collaborative? Doctors views on working in the NHS.* London: British Medical Association.

Breines, J. G. & Chen, S. (2012). Self-compassion increases self-improvement motivation. *Personality and Social Psychology Bulletin*, 38(9), 1133–1143.

Brocklehurst, P., Hardy, P., Hollowell, J., Linsell, L., Macfarlane, A., McCourt, C., Marlow, N., Miller, A., Newburn, M., Petrou, S., Puddicombe, D., Redshaw, M., Rowe, R., Sandall, J., Silverton, L. & Stewart, M. (2011). Perinatal and maternal outcomes by planned place of birth for healthy women with low risk pregnancies: The Birthplace in England national prospective cohort study. *BMJ*, 343(7840).

Brown, B. (2006). Shame resilience theory: A grounded theory study on women and shame. *Families in Society*, 87(1), 43–52.

Butterworth, T., Faugier, J. & Burnard, P. (1998). *Clinical supervision and mentorship in nursing* (2nd edn), ed. Tony Butterworth, Jean Faugier and Philip Burnard. Cheltenham: Stanley Thornes.

Cleary, M., Kornhaber, R., Thapa, D., West, S. & Visentin, D. (2018). The effectiveness of interventions to improve resilience among health professionals: A systematic review. *Nurse Educ. Today*, 71, 247–263.

Cook, K. & Loomis, C. (2012). The Impact of choice and control on women's childbirth experiences. *J Perinat Educ*, 21(3), 158–168.

Dahlberg, U. & Aune, I. (2013). The woman's birth experience: The effect of interpersonal relationships and continuity of care. *Midwifery*, 29(4), 407–415.

Dahlen, H. G. & Caplice, S. (2014). What do midwives fear? *Women Birth*, 27(4), 266–270.

Davis, D. L. & Homer, C. S. (2016). Birthplace as the midwife's work place: How does place of birth impact on midwives? *Women Birth*, 29(5), 407–415.

de Boer, J., Lok, A., Van't Verlaat, E., Duivenvoorden, H. J., Bakker, A. B. & Smit, B. J. (2011). Work-related critical incidents in hospital-based health care providers and the risk of post-traumatic stress symptoms, anxiety, and depression: A meta-analysis. *Soc Sci Med*, 73(2), 316–326.

Delgado, C., Upton, D., Ranse, K., Furness, T. & Foster, K. (2017). Nurses' resilience and the emotional labour of nursing work: An integrative review of empirical literature. *International Journal of Nursing Studies*, 70, 71–88.

Dev, V., Fernando, A. T., 3rd, Lim, A. G. & Consedine, N. S. (2018). Does self-compassion mitigate the relationship between burnout and barriers to compassion? A cross-sectional quantitative study of 799 nurses. *Int J Nurs Stud*, 81, 81–88.

DH (1993). *Report of the Expert Maternity Group: Changing childbirth (Cumberlege Report).* London: HMSO.

DH (2007). *Maternity Matters.* London: HMSO.

Duarte, J., Pinto-Gouveia, J. & Cruz, B. (2016). Relationships between nurses' empathy, self-compassion and dimensions of professional quality of life: A cross-sectional study. *International Journal of Nursing Studies*, 60, 1–11.

Ellis, A. (1994). *Reason and emotion in psychotherapy*. Secaucus, NJ: Lyle Stuart.

Everly, M. C. (2012). Facilitators and barriers of independent decisions by midwives during labor and birth. *J Midwifery Womens Health*, 57(1), 49–54.

Figley, C. R. (1995). *Compassion fatigue: Coping with secondary traumatic stress disorder in those who treat the traumatized.* New York: Brunner/Mazel.

Forbes, D., Fletcher, S., Parslow, R., Phelps, A., O'Donnell, M. & Bryant, R. (2012). Trauma at the hands of another: Longitudinal study of differences in the posttraumatic stress disorder symptom profile following interpersonal compared with non-interpersonal trauma. *J Clin Psychiatry*, 73(3), 372–376.

Francis, R. (2013). *Report of the Mid Staffordshire NHS Foundation Trust Public Inquiry.* London: The Stationery Office. Available online: https://webarchive.nationalarchives.gov.uk/20150407084949/www.midstaffspublicinquiry.com/sites/default/files/report/Executive%20summary.pdf [Accessed 1 August 2019].

Green, J. M. & Baston, H. A. (2003). Feeling in control during labor: Concepts, correlates, and consequences. *Birth*, 30(4), 235–247.

Hallam, J. L., Howard, C., Locke, A. & Thomas, M. (2016). Communicating choice: An exploration of mothers' experiences of birth. *Journal of Reproductive and Infant Psychology*, 34(2), 175–184.

Hammond, A., Foureur, M., Homer, C. S. E. & Davis, D. (2013). Space, place and the midwife: Exploring the relationship between the birth environment, neurobiology and midwifery practice. *Women and Birth*, 26(4), 277–281.

Hammond, A., Homer, C. S. E. & Foureur, M. (2017). Friendliness, functionality and freedom: Design characteristics that support midwifery practice in the hospital setting. *Midwifery*, 50, 133–138.

Hauck, Y., Lewis, L., Kuliukas, L., Butt, J. & Wood, J. (2016). Graduate midwives' perception of their preparation and support in using evidence to advocate for women's choice: A Western Australian study. *Nurse Educ Pract*, 16(1), 305–311.

Health Education England (2019) *Workforce Stress and the Supportive Organisation – A framework for improvement through reflection, curiosity and change.* London: HEE. Available online: www.hee.nhs.uk/sites/default/files/documents/Workforce%20Stress%20and%20the%20Supportive%20Organisation_0.pdf [Accessed 1 August 2019].

Healy, S., Humphreys, E. & Kennedy, C. (2016). Midwives' and obstetricians' perceptions of risk and its impact on clinical practice and decision-making in labour: An integrative review. *Women Birth*, 29(2), 107–116.

Healy, S., Humphreys, E. & Kennedy, C. (2017). A qualitative exploration of how midwives' and obstetricians' perception of risk affects care practices for low-risk women and normal birth. *Women Birth*, 30(5), 367–375.

Heffernan, M., Quinn Griffin, M. T., McNulty, S. R. & Fitzpatrick, J. J. (2010). Self-compassion and emotional intelligence in nurses. *International Journal of Nursing Practice*, 16(4), 366–373.

Hobbs, J. A. (2012). Newly qualified midwives' transition to qualified status and role: assimilating the 'habitus' or reshaping it? *Midwifery*, 28(3), 391–9.

Hodnett, E. (2002). Pain and women's satisfaction with the experience of childbirth: A systematic review*1. *American Journal of Obstetrics and Gynecology*, 186(5), S160–S172.

Hu, T., Zhang, D. & Wang, J. (2015). A meta-analysis of the trait resilience and mental health. *Personality and Individual Differences*, 76, 18–27.

Hunter, B. (2004). Conflicting ideologies as a source of emotion work in midwifery. *Midwifery*, 20(3), 261–272.

Hunter, B. (2005). Emotion work and boundary maintenance in hospital-based midwifery. *Midwifery*, 21(3), 253–266.

Hunter, B., Berg, M., Lundgren, I., Olafsdottir, O. A. & Kirkham, M. (2008). Relationships: The hidden threads in the tapestry of maternity care. *Midwifery*, 24(2), 132–137.

Hunter, B., Henley, J., Fenwick, J., Sidebotham, M. & Pallant, J. (2018). *Work, health and emotional lives of midwives in the United Kingdom: The UK WHELM study*. London: The Royal College of Midwives.

Hunter, B. & Warren, L. (2014). Midwives' experiences of workplace resilience. *Midwifery*, 30(8), 926–934.

Ishak, W. W., Kahloon, M. & Fakhry, H. (2011). Oxytocin role in enhancing well-being: A literature review. *Journal of Affective Disorders*, 130(1–2), 1–9.

Jackson, S. E. & Maslach, C. (1982). After-effects of job-related stress: Families as victims. *Journal of Organizational Behavior*, 3(1), 63–77.

Jordan, J. V. (2010). *Relational-cultural therapy.* Washington, DC: American Psychological Association.

Kirkup, B. (2015) .*The Report of the Morecambe Bay Investigation.* London: The Stationery Office. Available online: www.gov.uk/government/publications [Accessed 8 May 2019].

Kotter, J. P. & Heskett, J. L. (2008). *Corporate culture and performance.* New York: Free Press; Reprint edition (30 June 2008).

Kuliukas, L. J., Hauck, Y. C., Lewis, L. & Duggan, R. (2017). The woman, partner and midwife: An integration of three perspectives of labour when intrapartum transfer from a birth centre to a tertiary obstetric unit occurs. *Women and Birth*, 30(2), e125–e131.

Kuyken, W., Watkins, E., Holden, E., White, K., Taylor, R. S., Byford, S., Evans, A., Radford, S., Teasdale, J. D. & Dalgleish, T. (2010). How does mindfulness-based cognitive therapy work? *Behaviour Research and Therapy*, 48(11), 1105–1112.

Ledoux, K. (2015). Understanding compassion fatigue: understanding compassion. *J Adv Nurs*, 71(9), 2041–50.

Leinweber, J., Creedy, D. K., Rowe, H. & Gamble, J. (2017a). A socioecological model of post-traumatic stress among Australian midwives. *Midwifery*, 45, 7–13.

Leinweber, J., Creedy, D. K., Rowe, H. & Gamble, J. (2017b). Responses to birth trauma and prevalence of posttraumatic stress among Australian midwives. *Women Birth*, 30(1), 40–45.

Leinweber, J. & Rowe, H. J. (2010). The costs of 'being with the woman': Secondary traumatic stress in midwifery. *Midwifery*, 26(1), 76–87.

Love, B., Sidebotham, M., Fenwick, J., Harvey, S. & Fairbrother, G. (2017). "Unscrambling what's in your head": A mixed method evaluation of clinical supervision for midwives. *Women Birth*, 30(4), 271–281.

Luthar, S. S., Cicchetti, D. & Becker, B. (2000). The construct of resilience: A critical evaluation and guidelines for future work. *Child Development*, 71(3), 543–562.

Macbeth, A. & Gumley, A. (2012). Exploring compassion: A meta-analysis of the association between self-compassion and psychopathology. *Clinical Psychology Review*, 32(6), 545–552.

Manomenidis, G., Panagopoulou, E. & Montgomery, A. (2019). Resilience in nursing: The role of internal and external factors. *Journal of Nursing Management*, 27(1), 172–178.

Mautner, E., Stern, C., Deutsch, M., Nagele, E., Greimel, E., Lang, U. & Cervar-Zivkovic, M. (2013). The impact of resilience on psychological outcomes in women after preeclampsia: An observational cohort study. *Health and Quality of Life Outcomes*, 11.

McDonald, G., Jackson, D., Vickers, M. H. & Wilkes, L. (2016). Surviving workplace adversity: A qualitative study of nurses and midwives and their strategies to increase personal resilience. *Journal of Nursing Management*, 24(1), 123–131.

Meredith, L. S., Sherbourne, C. D., Gaillot, S. J., Hansell, L., Ritschard, H. V., Parker, A. M. & Wrenn, G. (2011). Promoting psychological resilience in the U.S. Military. *Rand Health Quarterly*, 1(2), 2.

Măirean, C. & Turliuc, M. N. (2013). Predictors of vicarious trauma beliefs among medical staff. *Journal of Loss and Trauma*, 18(5), 414–428.

Neff, K. (2003). Self-compassion: An alternative conceptualization of a healthy attitude toward oneself. *Self and Identity*, 2(2), 85–101.

NHS England (2016). *Better Births: Improving outcomes of maternity services in England – A five year forward view for maternity care.* London: NHS England. Available online: www.england.nhs.uk/wp-content/uploads/2016/02/national-maternity-review-report.pdf [Accessed 1 July 2019].

NHS England (2017) *A-EQUIP a model of clinical midwifery supervision.* London: NHS England. Available online: www.england.nhs.uk/wp-content/uploads/2017/04/a-equip-midwifery-supervision- model.pdf [Accessed 1 August 2019].

NHS England (2019). *Friends and Family Test.* London: NHS England. Available online: www.england.nhs.uk/publication/friends-and-family-test-data-june-2019/ [Accessed 8 August 2019].

NICE (2014). *Intrapartum care for healthy women and babies (CG190).* London: National Institute for Health and Care Excellence.

NMC (2009). *Standards for pre-registration midwifery education.* London: Nursing and Midwifery Council.

Nolte, A. G., Downing, C., Temane, A. & Hastings-Tolsma, M. (2017). Compassion fatigue in nurses: A metasynthesis. *J Clin Nurs*, 26(23–24), 4364–4378.

O'Connell, R. & Downe, S. (2009). A metasynthesis of midwives' experience of hospital practice in publicly funded settings: Compliance, resistance and authenticity. *Health (London)*, 13(6), 589–609.

Pezaro, S., Clyne, W., Turner, A., Fulton, E. A. & Gerada, C. (2016). 'Midwives Overboard!' Inside their hearts are breaking, their makeup may be flaking but their smile still stays on. *Women Birth*, 29(3), e59–66.

Porter, S., Crozier, K., Sinclair, M. & Kernohan, W. G. (2007). New midwifery? A qualitative analysis of midwives' decision-making strategies. *Journal of Advanced Nursing*, 60(5), 525–534.

Proctor, B. (1986) Supervision: A co-operative exercise in accountability. In M. Marken & M. Payne (eds), *Enabling and ensuring – supervision in practice*. Leicester, UK: National Youth Bureau, Council for Education and Training in Youth and Community Work.

Rice, H. & Warland, J. (2013). Bearing witness: Midwives experiences of witnessing traumatic birth. *Midwifery*, 29(9), 1056–1063.

Robertson, J. H. & Thomson, A. M. (2016). An exploration of the effects of clinical negligence litigation on the practice of midwives in England: A phenomenological study. *Midwifery*, 33, 55–63.

Rockliff, H., Gilbert, P., McEwan, K., Lightman, S. & Glover, D. (2008). A pilot exploration of heart rate variability and salivary cortisol responses to compassion-focused imagery. *Clinical Neuropsychiatry*, 5(3), 132–139.

Rowe, R. (2010). Local guidelines for the transfer of women from midwifery unit to obstetric unit during labour in England: a systematic appraisal of their quality. *Qual. Saf. Health Care*, 19(2), 90–94.

Ruotsalainen, J., Verbeek, J., Mariné, A. & Serra, C. (2015). Preventing occupational stress in healthcare workers. *Cochrane Database of Systematic Reviews* (4).

Sackett, D. L. (1997). Evidence-based medicine. *Seminars in Perinatology*, 21(1), 3–5.

Sandall, J., Soltani, H., Gates, S., Shennan, A. & Devane, D. (2015). Midwife-led continuity models versus other models of care for childbearing women. *Cochrane Database Syst Rev* (9), CD004667.

Savage, W. & Francome, C. (2007). British consultants' attitudes to caesareans. *Journal of Obstetrics and Gynaecology: The Journal of the Institute of Obstetrics and Gynaecology*, 27(4), 354–359.

Schroder, K., Jorgensen, J. S., Lamont, R. F. & Hvidt, N. C. (2016). Blame and guilt – a mixed methods study of obstetricians' and midwives' experiences and existential considerations after involvement in traumatic childbirth. *Acta Obstet Gynecol Scand*, 95(7), 735–745.

Seibold, C., Licqurish, S., Rolls, C. & Hopkins, F. (2010). 'Lending the space': Midwives' perceptions of birth space and clinical risk management. *Midwifery*, 26(5), 526–531.

Sheen, K., Spiby, H. & Slade, P. (2015). Exposure to traumatic perinatal experiences and posttraumatic stress symptoms in midwives: Prevalence and association with burnout. *Int J Nurs Stud*, 52(2), 578–587.

Sheppard, F., Stacey, G. & Aubeeluck, A. (2018). The importance, impact and influence of group clinical supervision for graduate entry nursing students. *Nurse Education in Practice*, 28, 296–301.

Sidebotham, M., Fenwick, J., Rath, S. & Gamble, J. (2015). Midwives' perceptions of their role within the context of maternity service reform: An appreciative inquiry. *Women and Birth*, 28(2), 112–120.

Sinclair, S., Raffin-Bouchal, S., Venturato, L., Mijovic-Kondejewski, J. & Smith-MacDonald, L. (2017). Compassion fatigue: A meta-narrative review of the healthcare literature. *Int J Nurs Stud*, 69, 9–24.

Smith, G. (1999). Resilience concepts and findings: Implications for family therapy. *Journal of Family Therapy*, 21(2), 154–158.

Symon, A. (2000). Litigation and defensive clinical practice: Quantifying the problem. *Midwifery*, 16(1), 8–14.

Thacker, S., Stroup, D. & Chang, M. (2001). Continuous electronic heart rate monitoring for fetal assessment during labor. *Cochrane Database of Systematic Reviews* (2).

Thompson, N. J., Fiorillo, D., Rothbaum, B. O., Ressler, K. J. & Michopoulos, V. (2018). Coping strategies as mediators in relation to resilience and posttraumatic stress disorder. *Journal of Affective Disorders*, 225, 153–159.

Vigna, A., Poehlmann-Tynan, J. & Koenig, B. (2018). Does self-compassion facilitate resilience to stigma? A school-based study of sexual and gender minority youth. *Mindfulness*, 9(3), 914–924.

Wahlberg, A., Andreen Sachs, M., Bergh Johannesson, K., Hallberg, G., Jonsson, M., Skoog Svanberg, A. & Hogberg, U. (2017). Self-reported exposure to severe events on the labour ward among Swedish midwives and obstetricians: A cross-sectional retrospective study. *Int J Nurs Stud*, 65, 8–16.

Waldenstrom, U., Hildingsson, I., Rubertsson, C. & Radestad, I. (2004). A negative birth experience: Prevalence and risk factors in a national sample. *Birth-Issues in Perinatal Care*, 31(1), 17–27.

Wallbank, S. (2013). Recognising stressors and using restorative supervision to support a healthier maternity workforce: A retrospective, cross-sectional, questionnaire survey. *Evidence Based Midwifery*, 11(1), 4–9.

Wendt, S., Tuckey, M. R. & Prosser, B. (2011) Thriving, not just surviving, in emotionally demanding fields of practice. *Health and Social Care in the Community*, 19(3), 317–325.

West, M., Eckert, R., Collins, B. & Chowla, R. (2017) *Caring to change How compassionate leadership can stimulate innovation in health care.* London: Kings Fund.

West, M. & Willis, D. (2015). *Are we supporting or sacrificing NHS staff?* London: Kings Fund.

West, M. A. & Dawson, J. F. (2012). *Employee engagement nhs performance.* London: Kings Fund. Available online: www.kingsfund.org.uk/sites/default/files/employee-engagement-nhs-performance-west-dawson-leadership-review2012-paper.pdf [Accessed 1 June 2019].

Yoshida, Y. & Sandall, J. (2013). Occupational burnout and work factors in community and hospital midwives: A survey analysis. *Midwifery*, 29(8), 921–926.

8 Using narratives to inform practice

Introduction

Gaining feedback from patients accessing healthcare has become an essential component of healthcare services in the UK (NHS England, 2019).Understanding and capturing how women and their families experience care across the whole pregnancy, birth and postnatal continuum can be challenging, as there are so many differing services to evaluate. The journey of a woman who has been diagnosed with gestational diabetes, for instance, will be different to a woman experiencing twins or an uneventful second pregnancy. Cultural differences, age and sexual orientation will all play a role in how women evaluate the services we provide; in addition, how and when feedback is obtained can affect its interpretation (Waldenström & Schytt, 2009). Quantitative satisfaction surveys that offer a numerical score can inform us if women are satisfied or dissatisfied with an area or process of care, but are often not then aggregated against the perceived importance to the woman (Sandin-Bojö et al, 2011). For women who have just given birth, the measure of satisfaction is susceptible to the 'halo effect' as the arrival of a healthy baby overshadows all other experiences (Simkin, 1992). In addition, women with no prior experience of maternity care tend to believe that the care they received is the norm: they have no other reference point on which to compare, and so in effect we are evaluating the 'status quo' (Teijlingen et al, 2003).

Listening to women and using narratives from birth afterthoughts sessions offer another opportunity to evaluate care. Often similar themes run through the multiple narratives, which afford us some insight into the lived experience of women accessing care, and to have an understanding of what it felt like and the impact. It adds a different dimension to the evaluation of care.

Perceived experience: does it still count?

As discussed earlier, memory is not a camera snapshot of an event. Time and spatial awareness can be blurred, as too the dialogue and intonation of the speech used by healthcare professionals. This can often be corrected or given context as part of the *reflect and reappraise* stage discussed in Chapter 4. There have been times when women have repeated a phrase used by a member of staff that is well known and seems innocuous; it is about understanding and accepting that even with the best intentions at that point for that woman, it was not helpful. Often it is not the actual phrase or words but the meaning that is subsequently attached to it by the woman. If a woman with symphysis pubis dysfunction, who has found lying down very uncomfortable since thirty-five weeks and has been awake and in pain with contractions for the last thirty-six hours is met by a busy midwife who says briskly 'just hop up here then' whilst patting the bed, the woman may attach the meaning 'she is being unkind'. The meaning attached to this comment then becomes a lens through which she views the episode of care and further interactions with staff. Given another context the phrase may not even be remembered. This example also leads back to the debate around caring for women within a continuity model: had she been met by a midwife who she knew and trusted, and already held in positive regard, would the scenario play out the same?

The other element that we must be careful not to lose sight of is that during a birth afterthoughts session, the meaning of the narrative is attributed by both the woman (narrator) and the midwife (listener). When listening to dialogue we also are subjected to the limitations and possibilities of being human (Fay, 1987), of not listening properly, and of misinterpreting what has been said and in making value judgements. It is also the listener that determines the value of the answer. For that reason it is useful in a birth afterthoughts session to clarify meaning rather than risk making assumptions, especially if it is going to be used as feedback to a healthcare professional. As Cardiff (2012) asserts, 'the truth within narratives is never absolute', because it cannot be valid for all people, in all societies and at all times. Every narrative is a negotiation about what reality was really like and we must appreciate how a woman chooses to tell her story and the aspects good and bad that she recalls (Shapiro, 2011). Instead of dissecting stories and looking for inaccuracies, it is useful to 'think with' rather than 'think about' stories as a form of empathic witnessing (Frank, 2015).

There are times when feedback requires immediate attention, either due to concerns with care or inappropriate language that has been used by a professional and this should be escalated appropriately and timely. However, the majority of narratives involve more subtle undertones and what we are interested in is how it made the woman *feel*. Depending on the context, feeding back 'she said you said' to an individual is not always helpful and is usually met with 'I would never say that'. What is more helpful is to talk through with the midwife a précised version of the woman, who she is, her journey and her experience, followed by a reflective discussion. If there is an actual line of dialogue this can be discussed but it has to be wrapped around the context of what was going on for that women at that point in time and a discussion around why she has attached so much meaning to the phrase. It is not about judging what is right or wrong. It is about understanding that how women subjectively experience care is complex and we all play a part. So the perceived experience of an individual is valid but it has to be appreciated and translated within that context. Used well it can support reflection in practice.

Critical reflection using narratives

As healthcare professionals, we make clinical decisions in a myriad of contexts and are often rewarded with an instant appraisal of our decision based on outcome, that is, a healthy baby, born in a good condition. For women worldwide, being safe in maternity care is more than physical safety and good-quality clinical care; women want improved communication, education, information, and respect from their providers as essential aspects of their experience (Renfrew et al, 2014). Learning from narratives offers contextual insights unique to that woman as an additional layer of reflection on which to base a modification or not, to the way we practice (Gilkison et al, 2016). It also allows us to reconnect with our own values and beliefs and understand how these shape our practice. As Gilkison (2016) asserts, 'knowledge and skills can be learned from lectures, textbooks and multimedia presentations, but the art of practice cannot be learned by simply absorbing information'. Hearing narratives offers a brief insight, a chance to 'walk in their shoes' and as such this can trigger feelings of empathy, described as sharing aspects of, or mirroring of, another's emotions (Jones & Ficklin, 2012), though exact definitions of empathy are still debated (Carlozzi et al, 2002) it is thought that as we hear narratives they trigger memories involving a similar situation and emotion or through socialisation processes we learn how emotions are experienced by individuals (Niedenthal, 2006). This then informs our reflection and learning from an incident.

Reflection is the way we learn from experience to generate new knowledge (Schon, 1983) and the analogy often used is of holding up a mirror to what we do. Reflective practice is a fusion of reflection, self-awareness and critical thinking (Eby, 2000) and ensures our practice is holistic and woman centred (Carter et al, 2018). In Scheffer and Rubenfeld's (2000) consensus statement on critical thinking, they list ten core components termed 'habits of the mind', including the ability to consider the whole situation (contextual perspective), seeking new knowledge and understanding (inquisitiveness), being receptive to divergent views and our own biases (open-mindedness), and self-evaluation for deeper understanding (reflection). This is a useful framework for critical reflection in practice.

These reflective accounts often deal with recurring themes, for instance communication, information, feeling a loss of control and perception of pain. These components are well evidenced as being important to how women appraise their birth experience (Henriksen et al, 2017; Hildingsson, 2015; Waldenström & Schytt, 2009).

Using narratives to mobilise change

Discussing narrative feedback and themes with healthcare professionals on a one-to-one basis or as part of a group discussion is one way to influence change and promote reflection. Some of the recurring themes, however, can be a used as a driver for getting larger scale change into practice. Knowledge transformation, whereby new knowledge is adopted into practice, is complex, takes time and is not automatically absorbed into practice (Grimshaw et al, 2012) by everyone at the same time. Even clinical guidelines which assimilate new evidence for use locally can take time within a unit to be implemented. In addition, not every aspect of practice is written down in a guideline or a standard operating procedure.

If we explore the area of 'skin to skin' as an example we would expect all midwives to understand that skin-to-skin contact equates to the baby being dried and placed naked on the mothers chest at or soon after birth, though not exclusively after birth. There is a growing evidence base to inform us that the duration of skin-to-skin holding is positively associated with exclusive breastfeeding (Bramson et al, 2010) and the increased levels of oxytocin during skin to skin may strengthen the mother's instinct to protect and care for her infant (Moore et al, 2016). It also supports thermoregulation of the newborn, maintaining a newborn's temperature post-birth (Safari & Moghaddam-Banaem, 2018). When skin to skin is not facilitated there is evidence that this can affect an infant's emotional and cognitive development in the long term (Flacking et al, 2012). In addition, we positively espouse the benefits of skin to skin during the pregnancy as it is woven throughout the UNICEF Baby Friendly Initiative (BFI) Accreditation standard 2:15, 'Support all mothers and babies to initiate a close relationship and feeding soon after birth' (UNICEF, 2012). In doing so, we create an expectation that it will happen, we place a value on its worth, whether intentional or not and as such women want it (Stevens et al, 2019) and expect it. Having created this expectation, what then happens when unplanned events occur, such as a woman being transferred to theatre for caesarean section or for a manual removal of placenta when skin to skin is not seen as the norm and is not written into the guideline?

Women who have a caesarean birth are less likely to experience skin-to-skin contact contact immediately after birth and all the associated benefits (Stevens et al, 2018; Zwedberg et al, 2015) even though their pre-birth expectation may have been that this would occur. The evidence also shows that women are more likely to experience breastfeeding difficulty and an early cessation of breastfeeding (Zanardo et al, 2010) so supporting skin to skin is an important component care. Midwives may understand the importance of skin to skin and actively facilitate it during births they attend at home or in hospital, but how does that same midwife negotiate and influence practice in obstetric theatre, and how easy is it to ensure the women they are caring for receive skin to skin in that setting? From experience, as reflected in the evidence, there are a different set of challenges and additional tasks that can take precedence over facilitating skin to skin in a theatre environment (Stevens et al, 2016; Stevens et al, 2018; Zwedberg et al, 2015). Getting the experience right in obstetric theatre is not solely down to the midwife; it is a team effort and as such any improvements need to be collectively owned. When the narratives from women expose this type of practice issue and we hear the effect it has had on their birth experience, then we need to look at wider service change and how narratives can shape those changes. In their narratives of obstetric theatre, women and their partners find it hard to quickly reappraise their surroundings, from the relaxed and friendly environment of a birth room to what feels like in the unwelcoming space of obstetric theatre. Common themes tend to report a disconnect from the process of birth, a sense that they are reduced to a body, a passive bystander and then a baby appears. This disconnect often continues in a woman's appraisal of her post-birth attachment journey. In theatre, women have an obstructed view during the process, so they are unable to see their baby being born. When the baby does not cry instantly, women become concerned quickly that something is wrong. Sometimes when a baby suddenly appears and is delivered prone to the chest it is hard for the mother to see her baby's face. When women are already feeling a disconnect from the birth process, they struggle to make sense of the speed and arrival of the baby, and so even when skin-to-skin contact is attempted it doesn't always feel positive.

> He was like a dead animal plonked on my chest ... he looked blue ... but I couldn't see his face ... I said 'is he ok'... then he was whisked away and no one said anything ... I started shaking and vomiting and then they bought him back tightly wrapped in blankets and said 'let's give him to dad to hold'... I had wanted skin to skin ... I had said I wanted skin to skin ...

No drama in our theatre: facilitating change in obstetric theatre

We have used the experience of obstetric theatre as described by women and their partners when they attended birth afterthoughts sessions to shape changes to practice in obstetric theatre (Brodrick & Baston, 2017). As part of the initiative we were passionate that the voices of women could be heard by a wider audience. We would actively encourage healthcare professionals to use narratives in this way as collectively they can be powerful (Phillips et al, 2016; Taylor & Hutchings, 2012). Our initiative was funded after a successful bid to the Getting Research into Practice (GRIP) funding stream supplied by National Institute Health Research Collaboration for Leadership in Applied Health Research and Care (NIHR, CLARC) which provides successful applicants with funds to support clinicians to mobilise knowledge and evidence and to make real changes to practice locally.

Exploring the complexities, challenges and opportunities in obstetric theatre requires sign-up from a multidisciplinary team. In the same way, we listen to women we must also listen to the narratives of our colleagues, working together to find a common understanding. One of the challenges we faced is that like other maternity units we had to understand the lived experience of the theatre staff, operating department assistants and nurses who staff our theatres. They operate in a world of sterility, procedures and checklists to maintain safe theatre practices and can be reluctant to give up rituals (Smith et al, 2009). The emotional and physicality of birth as midwives understand it, messy, unpredictable, euphoric, family centred, can feel very unfamiliar to theatre staff. In addition, they only see women for a snapshot in time. Stevens et al (2016) in their study describe this as a juxtaposition with staff recognising the emotional and social aspect of birth, yet also understanding the need for procedures with a theatre environment, leading to internal conflict within the staff members. Their voices, experience and concerns must be heard too to ensure collectively that we can seek some common ground. Central to this understanding are the narratives of women. As Smith et al (2009) argue, attention to tacit and implicit cultural factors, which underlie interprofessional working and communication in the theatres, is far more important than relying on protocols to change practice and behaviours. In addition, education has been shown to positively affect behavioural change in staff when initiating skin-to-skin contact in obstetric theatre (Berg & Hung, 2011). We identified shared agendas: relationship building takes time so it was important that regular meetings were scheduled to build trust and keep pace with the shifting clinical context. Membership of the project team was constantly reviewed and additional key personnel were invited as the need arose.

In our experience, making sustainable changes to practice requires an understanding of psychological and organisational theory which underlie behavioural change. This should then be wrapped around the context and conditions required for behaviour and practice change; this is illustrated by Michie et al's (2011) COM-B framework, which has been used successfully in influencing change in staff behaviour (Smith et al, 2019), including maternity (Hasted et al, 2016). The model recognises that *Behaviour* is affected by three core elements: *Capability, Opportunity* and *Motivation.* These drivers must be considered when looking at changing practice. Often, in our experience, improvement projects are positively championed by enthusiastic innovators with attention paid to motivating staff by sharing the benefits of a change. When we think about obstetric theatre, this can be quite disempowering; a midwife may be very well motivated to facilitate skin-to-skin contact and able to recite all the benefits, but what if her *opportunity* to do this is restricted because the woman needs to attend theatre for perineal suturing and skin to skin, when in these circumstances it has not traditionally been facilitated in theatre? Using the COM-B model it is possible to consider these points and plan for successful incorporation into the project implementation plan:

Capability: Do staff have the knowledge and understanding to facilitate skin to skin in theatre? Are they clear about the benefits of keeping mothers and babies together at all times? Are the able to challenge practice with their colleagues?

Motivation: Why change practice? How will it make a difference to women and their babies? Will it increase my workload? What if the baby gets cold?

Opportunity: Is it supported by colleagues? Is this how we do things here? Do we have the resources? Does the environment support this change in practice? Are the processes in place to keep things running smoothly in theatre?

Alongside the COM-B model we also utilised the Plan, Do, Study, Act model (Langley et al, 2009) which has been shown to be effective in a similar project looking at skin-to-skin contact in theatre (Brady et al, 2013).

We gathered intelligence by collecting the narratives and experiences from women and their partners to gain insight into their lived experience. These initial findings provided the focus for interviews with women and a baseline audit to enable the project team to measure success. To ensure the project could be embedded into practice, the funding bid included a project lead to work in theatres for one day a week to identify barriers to skin-to-skin contact, build relationships and work with staff to find solutions, providing mentorship and role modelling. The challenges and successes were fed back to the steering group, to ensure that the project was on target and further informed the spread strategy.

Women's narratives on obstetric theatre

The narratives from birth afterthoughts sessions highlighted a range of issues for women experiencing theatre. It is interesting to note that very few women attend birth afterthoughts following a planned caesarean section. Following previous practice changes, it was expected practice that skin-to-skin contact occurs during planned CS, although we had no evidence. As part of this project we conducted an audit of twenty-one planned cases occurring over a week and found that the majority of healthy babies were being placed on the resuscitaire to be dried with a mean separation time of 9.5 minutes and 52 per cent of partners left the mother to attend the resuscitaire. In addition, only 60 per cent of women could see their baby at all times in theatre. Follow-up face-to-face interviews revealed that most women could remember the name of the midwife, but none could recall the name of the surgeon or the anaesthetist, although they all said they were introduced to staff and felt welcome (Brodrick & Baston, 2017).

Many of the most poignant narratives were from women who needed theatre post-vaginal birth, including a woman requesting a caesarean section next time to avoid the risk of being separated again to undergo a manual removal of placenta (MROP). From experience is has been accepted practice in maternity services that for the purposes of suturing or manual removal of placenta the woman attends theatre alone post-birth, even in circumstances in which the mother is haemodynamically stable. See Case Study 8.1.

CASE STUDY 8.1 Hannah's experience

My labour was fine but I couldn't do the pushing part again and they said he was distressed so I had a ventouse … but it was fine … I was really looking forward to having skin to skin again and enjoying tea and toast … when he was born he was handed to me and the midwife was busily rubbing him with a towel, I felt overwhelmed … then the doctor asked the midwife for some help so she wrapped him up and handed him to my husband … lots of people came in the room and I was told my placenta was stuck … it all happened so quickly … I had to go to theatre … I remember the look on my husband's face as I was wheeled out … and I realised I was going alone … in theatre everyone was nice, the anaesthetist was asking me about names and the doctor was telling me about her daughter wanting to buy a skateboard … I laughed with everyone and chatted back … it all felt surreal … I had a newborn son somewhere, I remembering thinking I hadn't seen if all his fingers and toes were there … then I went into another room … the woman next to me was holding her baby and her husband was taking photos it seemed like hours had gone by.

I lost all that time with my son and it had a huge effect on the way I felt, on our bond, I knew it was different I just didn't feel the same as I did with my daughter. They kept saying every time is different you will learn to love him, and I did, but it is still not the same. We had always wanted three children but I said no for ages, he is six years old now and still our connection is not the same as my daughter. I don't think it ever will be. I will not take that risk again, I can't do that again, I want a caesarean then I know this time we will all stay together.

Narratives from partners left alone whilst the mother attends theatre often describe being 'left holding the baby' with concerns for their partner's health and trying to make sense of events.

> he was so small … fragile … I have never held a baby before … her blood was still on the floor … and we were all alone … I have never seen so much blood … they bought me tea … but I couldn't move … I just kept wishing things had been different.

Many partners reflected this anxiety of holding a newborn for the first time, alone in a room, frightened to move or change position. This reflects research which shows that in these circumstance fathers' feel anxious, fearful and abandoned (Etheridge & Slade, 2017). These accepted practices and the impact on women needed to be reflected back to staff in a non-judgemental way, to highlight and explore challenges in real practice and to work together for change. When we started to reflect on these practices and ask ourselves and others *why* this is the accepted norm, the answer was 'because we always have'.

Getting narratives heard: using forum theatre to reach a wider audience

Forum theatre was founded by the Brazilian theatre director Augustus Boal to enable interaction with the audience, and allows them to challenge and shape solutions to real practice scenarios (Boal, 2002). It has been used to explore challenging issues in healthcare such as end-of-life care (Tuxbury et al, 2012) and Alzheimer's (Kontos & Naglie, 2006) as well as in nursing and midwifery undergraduate training (Kemp, 2009; McClimens & Scott, 2007). Forum theatre can be delivered in a number of ways to highlight current evidence, local practice and the lived experience of women and partners. The enabling part of the methodology, however, lies in allowing the audience to provide solutions. From experience of listening to narratives used in conference presentations they can often illuminate hidden aspects of care and often add an additional poignancy and a chance to reflect on our values and beliefs. It invites us to connect in an engaging way and we can start to "see what we never noticed before, even though it was right in front of us' (Weber, 2008, p. 44). If it is done well, it invites the audience to reflect on personal understandings and how they are in the world, challenges dominant discourses and dissolve multidisciplinary silos (Mitchell et al, 2011). It can draw out the complexities of real-life practice settings, engaging the imagination and fostering compassion (Kontos & Naglie, 2006).

For this funded project, we were able to work with actors to develop two-hour interactive workshops. The narratives of women were delivered powerfully using monologues to the audience and then used to frame and re-enact theatre scenarios. Current evidence around the benefits of skin-to-skin contact were also woven through the different scenes. The workshop explored the experiences of staff, women and partners in theatre and highlighted staff tensions in a way that felt safe and non-threatening. It was a mix of humour, sadness and frustration played out in sketches and combined with optimism and the sense of a real opportunity. One of the most poignant portrayals was delivered by a midwife actor as a monologue to the audience based on real narratives from partners left alone 'holding the baby' and imagining the worst. Actually hearing real narratives and seeing the emotions of distress played out so realistically offers new and significant meaning to the lived experience of mothers and their partners (Taylor & Hutchings, 2012).

To support the facilitation of skin to skin in theatre, the central part of the workshop was a theatre scenario reflecting current practice and reflecting the themes from birth afterthoughts narratives, with a woman journeying from active labour in the midwifery led unit to emergency caesarean section in the obstetric theatre. The scenario is played a number of times with staff invited to 'clap' and stop whenever they saw a practice they wanted to comment on or change. Staff were asked to articulate how the woman might be feeling, using the first-person singular, for instance 'I am feeling scared and alone'; this sharing of thoughts and feelings can help make sense of the lived experience (Cardiff, 2012). As the scene is repeated, the audience is then handed control and given the opportunity to run the scenario differently, coming up with their own solutions, discussing and challenging each other with alternatives to facilitate family-centred care and skin-to-skin contact in theatre. This interactive approach to realising change enabled clinicians to trial behaviours and actions in a safe environment and to work together to overcome perceived organisational and environmental barriers. This has been shown in other studies to be fundamental to shifting cultural practice in obstetric theatre (Grassley & Jones, 2014; Stevens et al, 2016). Understanding the social and cultural context in which practice takes place is important to success. Rogers (2003) describes the term diffusion as the process by which a new practice is communicated over time among members of a social system. The success of an innovation then is dependent on social context, which is why even when the evidence base is strong it does not guarantee that the intervention will be accepted and adopted into practice (Dingfelder & Mandell, 2011). Enabling staff groups to work together and to explore different ways of working proved effective, with evaluations from the workshop reflecting findings from other studies whereby staff felt empowered to take action (Mitchell et al, 2011). In a systematic review of the diffusion of service innovations in healthcare, Greenhalgh et al (2004) discuss the need for innovations to be seen as complementing the organisational or professional values and norms (compatibility); to be broken down into manageable parts and easily assimilated into practice (complexity); the benefits need to be visible (observability); and adopters need to be able adapt and refine the innovation (reinvention). Exploring cultural change from the viewpoint of women, partners and staff though interactive engagement and working through solutions together supported the diffusion of incremental practice change with staff further discussing and questioning practice over time.

Central to the project's identity was the logo 'No Drama in Our Theatre', developed earlier in the process (Brodrick & Baston, 2017). This is used as a way to remind staff of the importance of getting it right for women experiencing obstetric theatre and continues to promote the work.

Conclusion

Listening to women's narratives of labour and birth offers us a unique insight into the lived experience of women and their partners. As we have discussed earlier in the book, how a woman remembers her birth and appraises her birth is not unidimensional; it is a complex journey interwoven within the subjective experience of birth. For women who feel unhappy with their care experience, it takes courage to come back and discuss a potentially upsetting experience and, as we listen, we too should show courage in owning the way in which the narratives are translated back into practice.

References

Berg, O. & Hung, K. (2011). Early skin-to-skin to improve breastfeeding after cesarean birth. *Journal of Obstetric Gynecologic and Neonatal Nursing*, 40, S18–S19.

Boal, A. (2002). *Games for actors and non-actors*. London: Routledge.

Brady, K. M., Bulpitt, D., Chiarelli, C. & Shepard, L. (2013). Skin-to-skin in the operating room—it takes a village. *Journal of Obstetric, Gynecologic, and Neonatal Nursing*, 42(s1), S42–S42.

Bramson, L., Lee, J. W., Moore, E., Montgomery, S., Neish, C., Bahjri, K. & Melcher, C. L. (2010). Effect of early skin-to-skin mother—infant contact during the first 3 hours following birth on exclusive breastfeeding during the maternity hospital stay. *Journal of Human Lactation*, 26(2), 130–137.

Brodrick, A. & Baston, H. (2017). Taking the drama out of obstetric theatre: Implementing change. *MIDIRS Midwifery Digest*, 27(4), 467–472.

Cardiff, S. (2012). Critical and creative reflective inquiry: Surfacing narratives to enable learning and inform action. *Educational Action Research*, 20(4), 605–622.

Carlozzi, A. F., Bull, K. S., Stein, L. B., Ray, K. & Barnes, L. (2002). Empathy theory and practice: A survey of psychologists and counselors. *The Journal of Psychology*, 136(2), 161–170.

Carter, A. G., Creedy, D. K. & Sidebotham, M. (2018). Critical thinking in midwifery practice: A conceptual model. *Nurse Education in Practice*, 33, 114–120.

Dingfelder, H. & Mandell, D. (2011). Bridging the research-to-practice gap in autism intervention: An application of diffusion of innovation theory. *Journal of Autism and Developmental Disorders*, 41(5), 597–609.

Eby, M. A. (2000) Understanding professional development. In A. Brechin, H. Brown, & M. A. Eby (eds), *Critical practice in health and social care*. London: Sage.

Etheridge, J. & Slade, P. (2017). "Nothing's actually happened to me": The experiences of fathers who found childbirth traumatic. *BMC Pregnancy and Childbirth*, 17(1), 80.

Fay, B. (1987). *Critical social science: Liberation and its limits.* Ithaca, NY: Cornell University Press.

Flacking, R., Lehtonen, L., Thomson, G., Axelin, A., Ahlqvist, S., Moran, V. H., Ewald, U. & Dykes, F. (2012). *Closeness and separation in neonatal intensive care. Acta Paediatrica*, 101(10), 1032–1037.

Frank, A. W. (2015). Asking the right question about pain: Narrative and phronesis. *British Journal of Pain*, 9(1), 209–225.

Gilkison, A., Giddings, L. & Smythe, L. (2016). Real life narratives enhance learning about the 'art and science' of midwifery practice. *Theory and Practice*, 21(1), 19–32.

Grassley, J. S. & Jones, J. (2014). Implementing skin-to-skin contact in the operating room following cesarean birth. *Worldviews on Evidence-Based Nursing*, 11(6), 414–416.

Greenhalgh, T., Robert, G., Macfarlane, F., Bate, P. & Kyriakidou, O. (2004). Diffusion of innovations in service organizations: Systematic review and recommendations. *Milbank Quarterly*, 82(4), 581–629.

Grimshaw, J., M., Eccles, M., P., Lavis, J. N., Hill, S. J. & Squires, J. E. (2012). Knowledge translation of research findings. *Implementation Science*, 7(1), 50.

Hasted, T., Stapleton, H., Beckmann, M. & Wilkinson, S. (2016). Clinician's attitudes to the introduction of routine weighing in pregnancy. *Journal of Pregnancy*, 2016(2016).

Henriksen, L., Grimsrud, E., Schei, B. & Lukasse, M. (2017). Factors related to a negative birth experience – a mixed methods study. *Midwifery*, 51, 33–39.

Hildingsson, I. (2015). Women's birth expectations, are they fulfilled? Findings from a longitudinal Swedish cohort study. *Women and Birth*, 28(2), e7–e13.

Jones, B. & Ficklin, L. (2012). To walk in their shoes: Recognising the expression of empathy as a research reality. *Emotion, Space and Society*, 5(2), 103–112.

Kemp, J. (2009). Exploring empowerment issues with student midwives using forum theatre. *British Journal of Midwifery*, 17(7), 438–439.

Kontos, P. C. & Naglie, G. (2006). Expressions of personhood in Alzheimer's: Moving from ethnographic text to performing ethnography. *Qualitative Research*, 6(3), 301–317.

Langley, G., Moen, R., Nolan, K., Nolan, T., Norman, C. & Provost, L. (2009). *The improvement guide: A practical approach to enhancing organizational performance* (2nd edn). San Francisco, CA: John Wiley & Sons.

McClimens, A. & Scott, R. (2007). Lights, camera, education! The potentials of forum theatre in a learning disability nursing program. *Nurse Education Today*, 27(3), 203–209.

Michie, S., van Stralen, M. M. & West, R. (2011). The behaviour change wheel: A new method for characterising and designing behaviour change interventions. *Implementation Science*, 6, 42.

Mitchell, G. J., Dupuis, S., Jonas-Simpson, C., Whyte, C., Carson, J. & Gillis, J. (2011). The experience of engaging with research-based drama: Evaluation and explication of synergy and transformation. *Qualitative Inquiry*, 17(4), 379–392.

Moore, E. R., Bergman, N., Anderson, G. C. & Medley, N. (2016). Early skin-to-skin contact for mothers and their healthy newborn infants. *Cochrane Database of Systematic Reviews* (11).

NHS England (2019). *Friends and Family Test.* London: NHS England. Available online: www.england.nhs.uk/publication/friends-and-family-test-data-june-2019/ [Accessed 8 August 2019].

Niedenthal, P. M. (2006). *Psychology of emotion: Interpersonal, experiential, and cognitive approaches.* New York and Hove: Psychology.

Phillips, H., Maw, H., Mee, S., Buckley, A. & Corless, L. (2016). How narratives can change nursing practice. *Nursing Times*, 112(17), 18–20.

Renfrew, M. J., McFadden, A., Bastos, M. H., Campbell, J., Channon, A. A., Cheung, N. F., Silva, D. R. A. D., Downe, S., Kennedy, H. P., Malata, A., McCormick, F., Wick, L. & Declercq, E. (2014). Midwifery and quality care: Findings from a new evidence-informed framework for maternal and newborn care. *The Lancet*, 384(9948), 1129–1145.

Rogers, E. M. (2003). *Diffusion of innovations* (5th edn). New York: Free Press, 2003.

Safari, K. & Moghaddam-Banaem, L. (2018). The effect of mother and newborn early skin-to-skin contact on initiation of breastfeeding, newborn temperature and duration of third stage of labor. *International Breastfeeding Journal*, 13(1).

Sandin-Bojö, A.-K., Kvist, L. J., Berg, M. & Wilde Larsson, B. (2011). What is, could be better. *International Journal of Health Care Quality Assurance*, 24(1), 81–95.

Scheffer, B. K. & Rubenfeld, M. G. (2000). A consensus statement on critical thinking in nursing. *The Journal of Nursing Education*, 39(8), 352–359.

Schon, D. A. (1983). *The reflective practitioner: How professionals think in action.* New York: Basic Books.

Shapiro, J. (2011). Illness narratives: Reliability, authenticity and the empathic witness. *Medical Humanities*, 37(2), 68.

Simkin, P. (1992). Just another day in a woman's life? Part 11: Nature and consistency of women's long-term memories of their first birth experiences. *Birth*, 19(2), 64–81.

Smith, A., Pope, C., Goodwin, D. & Mort, M. (2009). Teams, talk and transitions in anaesthetic practice, in L. Mitchell & R. Flin (eds), *Safer surgery: Analysing behaviour in the operating theatre.* Farnham, UK: Ashgate Publishing.

Smith, C., McNeill, A. & Kock, L. (2019). Exploring mental health professionals' practice in relation to smoke-free policy within a mental health trust: A qualitative study using the COM-B model of behaviour. *BMC Psychiatry*, 19.

Stevens, J., Schmied, V., Burns, E. & Dahlen, H. (2016). A juxtaposition of birth and surgery: Providing skin-to-skin contact in the operating theatre and recovery. *Midwifery*, 37, 41–48.

Stevens, J., Schmied, V., Burns, E. & Dahlen, H. G. (2018). Who owns the baby? A video ethnography of skin-to-skin contact after a caesarean section. *Women and Birth*, 31(6), 453–462.

Stevens, J., Schmied, V., Burns, E. & Dahlen, H. G. (2019). Skin-to-skin contact and what women want in the first hours after a caesarean section. *Midwifery*, 74, 140–146.

Taylor, A. M. & Hutchings, M. (2012). Using video narratives of women's lived experience of breastfeeding in midwifery education: Exploring its impact on midwives' attitudes to breastfeeding. *Maternal and Child Nutrition*, 8(1), 88–102.

Teijlingen, E., Hundley, V., Rennie, A., Graham, W. & Fitzmaurice, A. (2003). Maternity satisfaction studies and their limitations: "What is, must still be best". *Birth-Issue Perinat. Care*, 30(2), 75–82.

Tuxbury, J. S., Wall Mccauley, P. M. & Lement, W. (2012). Nursing and theatre collaborate: An end-of-life simulation using forum theatre. *The Journal of Nursing Education*, 51(8), 462–465.

UNICEF (2012). *UNICEF Guide to baby friendly initiative standards.* London: UNICEF. Available online: www.unicef.org.uk/wp-content/uploads/sites/2/2014/02/Baby_Friendly_guidance_2012.pdf [Accessed 1 August 2019].

Waldenström, U. & Schytt, E. (2009). A longitudinal study of women's memory of labour pain—from 2 months to 5 years after the birth. *BJOG: An International Journal of Obstetrics and Gynaecology*, 116(4), 577–583.

Weber, S. (2008). Visual images in research, in Cole, J. G. K. A. L. (ed.), *Handbook of the ARTS in qualitative research*. Thousand Oaks, CA: SAGE, 41–54.

Zanardo, V., Svegliado, G., Cavallin, F., Giustardi, A., Cosmi, E., Litta, P. & Trevisanuto, D. (2010). Elective cesarean delivery: Does it have a negative effect on breastfeeding? *Birth*, 37(4), 275–279.

Zwedberg, S., Blomquist, J. & Sigerstad, E. (2015). Midwives' experiences with mother–infant skin-to-skin contact after a caesarean section: 'Fighting an uphill battle'. *Midwifery*, 31(1), 215–220.

Index